W9-DDS-577

MedStudy®

4th Edition

Pediatrics Board Review Core Curriculum

Book 3 of 5

Topics in this volume:

The Fetus & Newborn

Genetics

Metabolic Disorders

Neurology

Authored by J. Thomas Cross, Jr., MD, MPH, FAAP, and Robert A. Hannaman, MD

NOTICE: Medicine and accepted standards of care are constantly changing. We at MedStudy do our best to review and include in this publication accurate discussions of the standards of care and methods of diagnosis. However, the author, the advisors, the editors, the publisher, and all other parties involved with the preparation and publication of this work do not guarantee that the information contained herein is in every respect accurate or complete. We recommend that you confirm the material with current sources of medical knowledge whenever considering presentations or treating patients.

A NOTE ON EDITORIAL STYLE: There is an ongoing debate in medical publishing about whether to use the possessive form that adds " 's " to the names of diseases and disorders, such as Lou Gehrig's disease, Klinefelter's syndrome, and others. We acknowledge there is not a unanimous consensus on this style convention, but we think it is important to be consistent in what style we choose. For this publication, we have dropped the possessive form. The *AMA Manual of Style*, *JAMA*, *Scientific Style and Format*, and *Pediatrics* magazine are among the publications now using the non-possessive form. MedStudy will use the non-possessive form in this Core Curriculum when the proper name is followed by a common noun. So you will see phrasing such as "This patient would warrant workup for Crohn disease." Possessive form will be used, however, when an entity is referred to solely by its proper name without a following common noun. An example of this would be "The symptoms are classic for Crohn's."

MEDSTUDY
P.O. Box 38148
Colorado Springs, Colorado 80937
(800) 841-0547

MedStudy®

4th Edition

Pediatrics Board Review Core Curriculum

The Fetus & Newborn

Authored by J. Thomas Cross, Jr., MD, MPH, FAAP, and Robert A. Hannaman, MD

Many thanks to

Daniel Polk, MD
Professor of Pediatrics
Northwestern University Medical School
Chief, Division of Hospital-Based Medicine
Children's Memorial Hospital
Division of Neonatology
Chicago, IL

and

Paul Catalana, MD, MPH
Professor of Clinical Pediatrics
Assistant Dean of Medical Education
University of South Carolina School of Medicine
Greenville, SC

The Fetus & Newborn Advisors

Table of Contents

The Fetus & Newborn

MORTALITY / MORBIDITY IN NEWBORNS 8-1
  COMMON TERMS 8-1
  FACTORS ASSOCIATED WITH NEONATAL MORTALITY 8-1
THE PLACENTA 8-2
  NOTE 8-2
  PLACENTAL DEVELOPMENT 8-2
  THE UMBILICAL CORD 8-2
  ABNORMALITIES OF THE PLACENTA 8-2
    Chorioamnionitis 8-2
    Placental Accreta 8-3
    Placental Percreta 8-3
    Placental Abruption 8-3
    Chorangioma 8-3
  ISSUES OF TWINS AND THEIR PLACENTAS 8-3
PRENATAL CARE 8-3
  "WELL-MOM" HEALTH 8-3
    Prenatal Visits 8-3
    Management of Group B Streptococcus Infection
      in Pregnancy 8-4
  PRETERM COMPLICATIONS 8-4
    Overview 8-4
    Premature Rupture of Membranes 8-5
    Preeclampsia 8-5
    Diabetes Mellitus 8-6
  ASSESSING FETAL HEALTH 8-6
    Fundal Height 8-6
    Ultrasound Imaging and Biometry 8-6
    Nonstress Testing 8-6
    Biophysical Profile 8-6
    Contraction Stress Test 8-6
    Fetal Heart Rate Monitoring 8-6
    Fetal Heart Rate Patterns 8-7
CESAREAN SECTION (C-SECTION) 8-9
OPERATIVE VAGINAL DELIVERY 8-9
FETAL-TO-NEWBORN TRANSITIONS 8-9
    Circulatory Transition After Birth 8-9
    Respiratory Transitions 8-11
    Glucose Transitions 8-11
    Water Balance 8-11
THE DELIVERY ROOM 8-11
  APGAR 8-11
  DELIVERY ROOM RESUSCITATION 8-11
    Overview 8-11
    Drugs 8-12
THE NEWBORN EXAMINATION 8-12
  OVERVIEW 8-12
  GESTATIONAL AGE / SIZE 8-13
    Sanity Break 8-14
    Back to Work 8-14
  CRYING IN THE NEWBORN 8-14
  TEMPERATURE 8-14
  SKIN 8-14
  THE HEAD 8-15
    Shape 8-15
    Fontanelles 8-15
    Craniosynostosis 8-15
    Caput Succedaneum 8-16
    Cephalohematoma 8-16
    Subgaleal Hemorrhage 8-16
    Skull Fractures 8-16
    Intracranial Bleeding 8-17

EYES 8-17
EARS 8-17
NOSE 8-18
MOUTH 8-18
NECK 8-18
CHEST 8-19
LUNGS 8-19
HEART 8-19
ABDOMEN 8-20
GENITALIA 8-20
ANUS 8-21
SPINAL COLUMN 8-21
EXTREMITIES 8-21
NEUROLOGICAL EXAM 8-22
  Mental Alertness 8-22
NEONATAL PROPHYLAXIS 8-22
  EYE PROPHYLAXIS 8-22
  VITAMIN K 8-23
  HEPATITIS B 8-23
  CORD CARE 8-23
  CIRCUMCISION 8-23
NEONATAL SCREENING 8-23
  GLUCOSE 8-23
  HEMATOCRIT 8-23
  BLOOD TYPE 8-23
  INBORN ERRORS OF METABOLISM /
    HEMOGLOBINOPATHIES 8-23
  HEARING 8-24
    Screening 8-24
  TOXIC SUBSTANCES / ILLICIT DRUGS 8-24
MULTIPLE BIRTHS 8-24
  EPIDEMIOLOGY 8-24
  PRENATAL ASSESSMENT 8-24
  DELIVERY AND PERINATAL PROBLEMS 8-24
SMALL FOR GESTATIONAL AGE (SGA) 8-24
DIABETES IN PREGNANCY 8-25
RESPIRATORY DISEASES OF THE NEWBORN 8-26
  RESPIRATORY DISTRESS SYNDROME
    HYALINE MEMBRANE DISEASE 8-26
  TRANSIENT TACHYPNEA OF THE NEWBORN 8-27
  PERSISTENT PULMONARY HYPERTENSION
    OF THE NEWBORN (PPHN) 8-27
  MECONIUM ASPIRATION 8-28
  PNEUMOTHORAX AND PNEUMOMEDIASTINUM 8-28
  PULMONARY HEMORRHAGE IN THE NEWBORN 8-29
  INTERSTITIAL PULMONARY FIBROSIS
    (WILSON-MIKITY SYNDROME) 8-29
  GROUP B STREPTOCOCCUS PNEUMONIA 8-29
PATENT DUCTUS ARTERIOSUS 8-30
GASTROINTESTINAL DISORDERS IN NEWBORNS 8-31
  MECONIUM PLUGS 8-31
  MECONIUM ILEUS 8-31
  NECROTIZING ENTEROCOLITIS 8-32
  HYPERBILIRUBINEMIA (NEWBORN JAUNDICE) 8-32
    Overview 8-32
    Treatment 8-34
    Kernicterus 8-34
    Treatment of Hyperbilirubinemia 8-34
BLOOD DISORDERS IN THE NEWBORN 8-36
  ERYTHROBLASTOSIS FETALIS 8-36

MORTALITY / MORBIDITY IN NEWBORNS

COMMON TERMS

Let's begin by defining common terms that will be on the ABP (American Board of Pediatrics) exam. Most of these terms are derived from the AAP (American Academy of Pediatrics) and ACOG (American College of Obstetricians and Gynecologists).

Live Birth: The complete "expulsion or extraction" from the mother of a product of human conception. The length of the pregnancy doesn't matter, as long as the baby breathes or shows "evidence of life"—a beating heart, pulsation of the umbilical cord, or definite movement of voluntary muscles. These life-evident criteria apply with or without the cutting of the umbilical cord, and whether or not the placenta is attached. Note: By accepted definition, "heartbeats" are discerned from "transient cardiac contractions" and "respirations" from "fleeting respiratory efforts or gasps."

Birth Weight: The weight of a neonate determined as soon as possible after delivery. Express it to the nearest gram.

Gestational Age: The number of weeks in a pregnancy since the first day of the last normal menstrual period.

Appropriate for Gestational Age (AGA): An infant with a birth weight that is between the 10th and 90th percentiles for the given gestational age.

Small for Gestational Age (SGA): An infant with a birth weight < 10th percentile for the given gestational age.

Large for Gestational Age (LGA): An infant with a birth weight > 90th percentile for the given gestational age.

Low Birth Weight (LBW): An infant whose birth weight is < 2,500 grams, regardless of gestational age.

Preterm: An infant born before the last day of the 37th week (259th day) of gestation. Or more simply—born before the 38th week of gestation!

Term: An infant born between the first day of the 38th week of gestation (260th day) and the end of the last day of the 42nd week (294th day) of gestation.

Post-term: An infant born on or after the first day of the 43rd week (the 295th day) of gestation.

Fetal Death: The opposite of "live birth"—a death that occurs before the infant is fully "expelled" or "extracted." By definition, there can be no "evidence of life," as described above relative to "live birth." Note: This definition by AAP/ACOG does not include "induced termination of pregnancy or abortion."

Infant Death: A death that occurs at any time from birth up to, but not including, 1 year of age (includes a death at 364 days, 23 hours, 59 minutes, 59 seconds; you get the picture here).

Perinatal Death: A death occurring between the 28th week of gestation and the 28th day of life.

Infant Mortality Rate: Expressed as the number of deaths per 1,000 live births.

FACTORS ASSOCIATED WITH NEONATAL MORTALITY

Race: On the sole criterion of race, mortality rates for infants are highest for African-Americans, followed by Native Americans, Caucasians, and finally, Asians and Pacific Islanders. However, the highest mortality for any multiple criteria group is seen in Caucasian infants weighing < 500 grams. This is one of those trick questions: Which race has the highest infant mortality rate? African-Americans. Which specific group has the highest mortality rate? Caucasian infants < 500 grams.

Maternal Factors: Prenatal care delayed until after the first trimester is associated with higher infant mortality rates. Also, infants born to teens, women > 40 who did not complete high school, unmarried women, women with underlying disease (chronic hypertension, autoimmune disease, diabetes mellitus), and smokers have higher mortality rates.

Sex: Male infants have higher mortality rates than female infants.

Multiple Births: Multiple gestations have higher mortality rates, accounting for > 25% of deliveries with birth weight < 1,500 grams! The availability of newer infertility treatments has brought about a huge increase in multiple gestations.

Preterm Infants: Although the relevant factors are frequently unknown, preterm infants have higher mortality rates.

Known risk factors for prematurity include:
• Placental bleeding (placenta previa, abruptio placentae)
• Uterine abnormalities (bicornate uterus, incompetent cervix)
• Cocaine abuse
• Maternal chronic diseases
• Premature rupture of membranes
• Chorioamnionitis
• Bacterial vaginosis
• Congenital abnormalities
• Polyhydramnios
• Group B streptococcus
• Sexually transmitted diseases (herpes, syphilis)
• Periodontal disease

Note: 10% of births are premature, but this 10% is responsible for > 65% of infant mortality/morbidity; 15% of infant deaths are due to prematurity/low birth weight.

Survival has improved markedly for infants with extremely low birth weight (< 1,500 grams), increasing to ~ 85%. For infants weighing < 500 grams, however, the survival rate is still 11–15%. Those who survive still have high morbidity, with chronic lung disease and intracranial hemorrhages being most common.

For preterm infants specifically, there are several independent risk factors for increased mortality:
• Male sex
• 5-minute APGAR < 4
• Lack of antenatal steroids
• Persistent bradycardia at 5 minutes

notes | Blue Baby |

Cardiac: generally nl WOB (except TAPVR)   Resp: ↑WOB
    Truncus—maybe↓
    Transpo
    Tetralogy
    Tricuspid atresia
    TAPVR
    Pulm valve stenosis
    Pulm artery stenosis

- Hypothermia
- Intrauterine growth restriction (IUGR)

Intrauterine Growth Restriction (IUGR): IUGR is present when a fetus is noted to be at < 5th percentile of growth for gestational age. The most common factors associated with IUGR include maternal hypertension and vascular disease associated with diabetes mellitus, malnutrition, and smoking. Alcohol use is also a common cause of microcephaly. Fetal growth may be compromised by infection, primordial dwarfing syndromes, chromosomal anomalies, and congenital malformation syndromes.

Congenital Malformation: This is the leading cause of infant death in the U.S., accounting for ~ 25% of infant mortality!

Respiratory Distress Syndrome: Once one of the leading causes of infant death, this syndrome now causes < 5% of infant deaths. This reduction primarily is due to the use of surfactant therapy and antenatal steroids. Cesarean section rates have also increased markedly in the low-birth-weight group, as have delivery room intubations.

Note: Even though mortality rates have decreased for low-birth-weight infants over the past 20 years, morbidity rates have not changed much for certain complications, such as chronic lung disease, intracranial bleeds, and retinopathy of prematurity.

THE PLACENTA

NOTE

We'll now review the development of this interesting organ—an organ so interesting, in fact, that an entire journal is devoted to it, titled, interestingly enough, *Placenta*.

PLACENTAL DEVELOPMENT

At ~ day 6, the embryo, at this stage called a "blastocyst," finishes its trip through the fallopian tube and "invades" the endometrium. The outer shell of the blastocyst is the trophoblast, which makes contact with the endometrium and covers the entire placenta. The trophoblast cells invade the maternal blood vessels and cause blood to leak into the space between cells. This process forms lacunae that become the intervillous space. The shell is composed of placental villi and membranes. The trophoblast becomes the barrier between mother and fetus. The outer part of the trophoblast is called the syncytium, which makes direct contact with the mother. Because it does not have major histocompatibility antigens, the syncytium does not react to, nor is it recognized by, the mother's body as "foreign." The syncytium is the means by which the fetus will get nutrients, oxygen, and water from the mother; it also is the means by which the fetus excretes wastes into the maternal bloodstream.

When developed, the placenta has an innermost surface called the amnion—a thin epithelial layer on top of connective tissue. The amnion is avascular and attached to the chorion, a tough membrane that carries the fetal blood vessels from the umbilical cord insertion across the placenta to the villous "ramifications." At ~ 12 weeks, the true (discoid) placenta begins to demarcate at the old embryonic pole. The placenta is attached by villi to the decidua, directly overlaying maternal arterioles. The other villi atrophy and disappear entirely by 16–18 weeks. The arterioles empty into the intervillous space so that maternal blood circulates around and through the latticework of villi, draining out through 2 or 3 venous sinuses. Usually, 1 artery will supply a single villous cotyledon (essentially a group of villi), which is then drained by 1 vein. A mature placenta will have anywhere from 10 to 20 cotyledons. Each cotyledon has a maternal artery that provides blood to the center. The fetal arteries then cross over the veins on the placental surface. Nutrients move from maternal blood to the intervillous space, across the trophoblast cells, through the fibrous core of the villus, and finally, through the endothelial cells of the fetal capillaries to the fetal blood. This is called a "hemochorial" placenta—maternal blood is in apposition to fetal chorionic or trophoblastic tissue.

THE UMBILICAL CORD

The umbilical cord contains 2 arteries and 1 vein. The cord usually implants directly on the placental surface; but in 1% of pregnancies, it will insert onto the membranes—a condition associated with growth retardation, and also frequently marked by the presence of only 1 artery. Term umbilical cords measure 55 cm in length. Shorter cords (< 40 cm) are rare and result in fetal morbidity, such as amnionic bands or muscular disorders. By contrast, longer cords are common, and they can form knots, prolapse, or entwine the fetus. The most common umbilical abnormality is the condition of having only 1 artery. 40% of these infants will die or have a major congenital abnormality; trisomy 18 is one of the most frequent abnormalities. Some authorities recommend renal ultrasonography in all infants with a single umbilical artery. The other 60% of infants with 1 umbilical artery generally have no problems. Note for the Board exam: If the question presents a child with a single umbilical artery, make sure you do a careful search for congenital anomalies.

ABNORMALITIES OF THE PLACENTA

Chorioamnionitis

Chorioamnionitis is infection of the amniotic fluid. Textbooks most commonly report this as occurring at 20–30 weeks; preterm chorioamnionitis is associated with preterm birth and subsequent developmental abnormalities. However, most neonatologists report increased experience with chorioamnionitis in term pregnancies that are complicated by prolonged (≥ 18 hours) rupture of membranes. Chorioamnionitis is almost always an ascending infection, unless it follows an amniocentesis. Fetal infection is most commonly caused by group B streptococcus, *Escherichia coli*, and *Listeria monocytogenes*.

notes

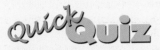

1) Which race has the highest infant mortality in the U.S.?
2) Which race/birth weight group has the highest infant mortality in the U.S.?
3) What maternal factors are associated with higher neonatal mortality?
4) Which sex has higher mortality rates?
5) For preterm infants, what independent risk factors are associated with increased mortality?
6) What is the leading cause of infant death in the U.S.?
7) How many arteries and veins does the normal umbilical cord contain?
8) If a newborn presents with a single umbilical artery, what should you do?
9) Define placental abruption.
10) Which types of twins have diamnionic, monochorionic placentas?
11) Which type of placenta is usually associated with fraternal twins?

Placental Accreta

Placental accreta develops when the uterus lacks normal decidua because of previous trauma, such as in curettage, myomectomy, or C-section.

Placental Percreta

Placental percreta develops when the placenta penetrates the scars in placental accreta, resulting in serious hemorrhage.

Placental Abruption

Placental abruption develops when a firm (organized) layer of blood forms after a retroplacental hemorrhage.

Choriangioma

Choriangioma arise from fetal villous circulation. They can become large, interfere with fetal circulation, and cause heart failure and hydrops.

ISSUES OF TWINS AND THEIR PLACENTAS

Multiple gestations: The placenta can be the clue to the origins of the babies! Placentas may be fused or separate. The membrane relationship may be monochorionic or dichorionic.

Monochorionic membranes are thin and translucent. At delivery, these membranes can be separated easily and show a single, chorionic surface that covers the villous tissue. This formation is referred to as diamnionic, monochorionic twin placentas. It is seen in monozygotic identical twins, when there is initially only 1 ovum before division.

Dichorionic twins are composed of 2 amnionic and 2 chorionic layers. It is difficult to separate these membranes. These placentas are diamnionic, dichorionic, and are usually associated with fraternal twins. Note: Identical twins could also have separate diamnionic, dichorionic placentas, provided that the twins separated early, before the formation of the chorionic cavity (i.e., before day 3).

Another issue in twins: When an artery on one twin supplies the cotyledon that is then drained by a vein into the other twin, the development of twin-to-twin transfusions can occur. One twin may develop polycythemia, while the other has anemia. This can escalate to CHF and hydrops in the recipient twin and decreased amnionic fluid volumes ("stuck twin") in the donor. This condition now can be treated prenatally by the use of a laser to obliterate the connection!

PRENATAL CARE
"WELL-MOM" HEALTH

Prenatal Visits

A basic regimen for the first prenatal visit should include the following:
1) Determine the first day of the last menstrual period to date the pregnancy.
2) Do a complete history and physical examination, including a pelvic exam.
3) Conduct laboratory testing:
   ◦ Urine for protein, glucose, and bacteriuria
   ◦ CBC
   ◦ VDRL or RPR
   ◦ Rubella antibodies
   ◦ Hepatitis B surface antigen
   ◦ Blood type and Rh
   ◦ Red cell antibodies
   ◦ Consider testing for GC, *Chlamydia*, and HIV if at increased risk
4) Education about nutrition, risk factors, and what to expect during the pregnancy.

Schedule and purposes for visits:
• 6–8 weeks gestation: See above for actions to take.
• 10–14 weeks: Check fetal heart tones.
• 16–20 weeks: Blood work for neural tube defects and chromosomal abnormalities—high alpha-fetoprotein (AFP) levels are often associated with neural tube defects, low AFP levels with trisomy 21, trisomy 13, and trisomy 18.
• 18–20 weeks: Ultrasound (U/S), if indicated.
• 22–26 weeks: Routine return visit.
• 28 weeks: Glucose tolerance test, repeat CBC, and evaluate for Rh immune globulin.
• 32 weeks, 36 weeks, and weekly thereafter: Routine return visits.

notes

Tachycardia

Sinus or SVT:
Sepsis
Hypovolemia
Hyperthyroid
- Mom ₹ Grave's ₹
IgG crosses placenta

If circulatory compromise, treat...
Vagal ~~~~: gag
ice to face
adenosine

Congenital hypothyroidism
hyperbili
low glucose
SGA

glandular: ↑TSH, ↓fT4

central: ↓TSH, ↓fT4
worry about pan-hypopit

Management of Group B Streptococcus Infection in Pregnancy

Group B streptococcus (GBS) remains a leading cause of neonatal infection, despite growing knowledge and application of CDC preventive guidelines issued in the 1990s. Guidelines were initially published in 1996, and updated in August 2002, for the prevention of perinatal GBS disease in pregnancy.

Changes in the 2002 guidelines:
- Do universal prenatal screening for vaginal and rectal GBS of all pregnant women between 35 and 37 weeks gestation.
- Discontinue recommending routine, intrapartum, antibiotic prophylaxis for GBS-colonized women undergoing planned C-section who have not begun labor, or have not had rupture of membranes.
- Institute antibiotic therapy in infants born following maternal intrapartum chorioamnionitis, after CBC and culture are obtained; treat until cultures are sterile x 48 hours.

Existing guidelines that remain unchanged:
- Penicillin (PCN) is the first-line agent for intrapartum antibiotic prophylaxis, with ampicillin as an alternative.
- Manage women whose culture results are unknown at the time of delivery, according to a risk-based approach: delivery < 37 weeks, membranes ruptured ≥ 18 hours, temperature ≥ 100.4° F.
- Women within 5 weeks of delivery who have negative vaginal and rectal cultures for GBS do not require intrapartum antimicrobial prophylaxis, even if the above obstetrical risk factors are present.
- Give intrapartum antimicrobial prophylaxis for women with GBS bacteriuria at any time during the current pregnancy or for women who previously gave birth to an infant with GBS disease, whether currently colonized or not.
- In the absence of GBS urinary tract infection, do not use antimicrobial agents before the intrapartum period to treat asymptomatic GBS colonization.

So the algorithm to follow is:
Do vaginal/rectal GBS screening cultures on all pregnant women at 35–37 weeks gestation, and prophylax them if the culture is positive (unless she is going to have a C-section, has not had active labor, and the membranes are intact).
Also prophylax the following women:
- Previously gave birth to an infant with invasive GBS disease
- GBS bacteriuria confirmed during the pregnancy
- Unknown GBS status (culture wasn't done or incomplete/unknown results) and any of the following 3 are present:

    Delivery is < 37 weeks
    Membrane rupture is ≥ 18 hours
    Intrapartum temperature is ≥ 100.4° F

Do not prophylax these women:
- Previous pregnancy with a positive GBS culture (unless the current pregnancy is also positive).
- Planned C-section in the absence of labor and with intact membranes (regardless of whether cultures are positive or negative).
- Cultures are negative at GBS screening.

What do you do if Mom needs prophylaxis?
- PCN G 5 million units IV x 1; then 2.5 million units IV q 4 hours until delivery (ampicillin is acceptable with 2g x 1 then 1 g q 4)
- If PCN-allergic:
  ◦ Low risk of anaphylaxis: cefazolin 2 g IV x 1, then 1 g IV q 8 hours until delivery
  ◦ High risk of anaphylaxis and the GBS is sensitive to clindamycin or erythromycin: use clinda or erythro
  ◦ High risk of anaphylaxis and the GBS is resistant to clinda/erythro, or sensitivities weren't done: use vancomycin

What about with preterm labor < 37 weeks?
- If no culture was done: First obtain vaginal/rectal GBS cultures and initiate IV PCN; if no growth in 48 hours, stop PCN; otherwise, continue PCN.
- If mother is known GBS+: Start PCN IV for minimum of 48 hours; continue prophylaxis until delivery. If delivery has not occurred by 4 weeks, repeat vaginal/rectal GBS culture and manage the patient, based on results of repeat GBS culturing.
- If mother is known GBS–: No prophylaxis is indicated.

Okay, now what about the neonate?
If the mother was given intrapartum antibiotics appropriately: see Figure 8-1—Algorithm for Management of Baby Born to Mom with GBS Prophylaxis (Note: Applies only to asymptomatic mothers and babies.)

PRETERM COMPLICATIONS

Overview

Preterm labor is defined as the onset of regular uterine contractions, producing changes in the cervix, at < 37 weeks gestation. The highest risk factor for preterm delivery is having a history of a previous preterm delivery.
Interventions currently consist of bed rest and various tocolytic agents. Tocolytic drugs, however, are not without side effects, and none has been shown to be superior to others. Preterm labor is so over-diagnosed that it is difficult to do well-controlled studies with these agents. In fact, placebo is shown to be 50% effective!
Always be aware of mothers with "incompetent cervix." This is due to cervical tissue that has simply matured too early, before term. It is usually seen only in mothers who have a prior history of this condition; it is difficult to diagnose in the nulliparas. If identified, a cerclage (placement of a ring/loop

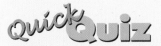

and 3rd trimesters. Once preeclampsia is identified, the woman needs to be followed carefully for any of these signs:
- Systolic BP ≥160 mmHg or diastolic BP ≥ 110 mmHg
- Proteinuria > 5 grams in 24 hours or ≥ 3+ on dipstick
- Oliguria < 500 mL/24 hours
- Visual or mental status changes
- Pulmonary edema or cyanosis
- Epigastric or upper abdominal pain
- Liver function abnormalities
- Thrombocytopenia (< 100,000 platelets/mm^3)

Any of these signs indicate "severe" preeclampsia, and delivery should be initiated quickly by induction or C-section. Proper treatment of the mother is paramount. Usually, BP is controlled with labetalol or hydralazine. Give magnesium sulfate to prevent seizures. Outcome for the infant in these cases is usually favorable, with the pressing issues being those related to prematurity.

For the Boards, remember the "HELLP" syndrome, characterized by hemolysis, elevated liver enzyme levels and a low platelet count. The pathogenesis of this obstetric complication is unclear, but it may be a variant of preeclampsia. Early diagnosis is critical because morbidity and mortality rates are

around the incompetent cervix) offers a solution, as does a stitch around the cervix to keep it closed.

Premature Rupture of Membranes

Premature rupture of membranes (PROM) is usually idiopathic, although infection or premature opening of the internal cervical os is a speculative cause. Know the following:

If PROM occurs at term or at 36–38 weeks gestation, evaluate the mother by speculum examination; check the fetus with fetal heart rate (FHR); and discern the fetal presentation. Most obstetricians proceed with induction.

At 34–36 weeks gestation, newborn morbidity is very low, and PROM is usually treated the same as at term.

At 32–33 weeks gestation, when pulmonary maturity is less likely, PROM management is controversial. Some obstetricians perform an amniocentesis to test for pulmonary maturity, while others allow simple bed rest with steroid therapy to induce pulmonary maturity. A 48-hour course of IV ampicillin and erythromycin followed by 5 days of amoxicillin and erythromycin is recommended during expectant management.

At < 28 weeks gestation, some obstetricians institute tocolysis, even with active contractions after the steroid therapy is started.

Note: If infection is diagnosed in conjunction with PROM, all of the above is invalid, and the baby is delivered as quickly as possible because the risk of serious fetal infection is directly proportional to the length of time between rupture of membranes and delivery.

Preeclampsia

Preeclampsia occurs in 3–7% of pregnancies. The etiology is unknown. Preeclampsia usually is identified early by monitoring blood pressure and urine protein during the late 2nd

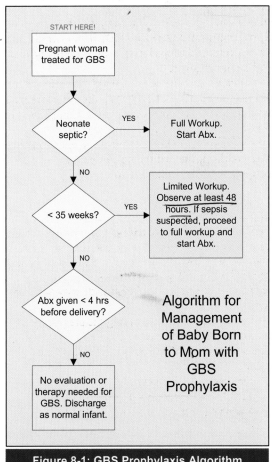

Figure 8-1: GBS Prophylaxis Algorithm

START HERE!

Pregnant woman treated for GBS

Neonate septic? — YES → Full Workup. Start Abx.

NO

< 35 weeks? — YES → Limited Workup. Observe at least 48 hours. If sepsis suspected, proceed to full workup and start Abx.

NO

Abx given < 4 hrs before delivery?

NO

No evaluation or therapy needed for GBS. Discharge as normal infant.

Algorithm for Management of Baby Born to Mom with GBS Prophylaxis

notes

as high as 25%. A positive D-dimer test may be an early identifier of patients with preeclampsia at risk of progression to HELLP syndrome. Treatment is supportive, including seizure prophylaxis and control of hypertension.

Diabetes Mellitus

Although pregnancy outcomes are excellent today with good management of maternal diabetes, there is still a higher frequency of congenital anomalies in these infants, even with good glucose control in the mother. The incidence of malformations is related to the degree of hyperglycemia prior to conception. Mothers should keep fasting blood sugars at 80–100 mg/dL, and keep 1-hour, post-meal values at 100–140 mg/dL. Before diabetic women become pregnant, they should have a glycosylated hemoglobin (HbA$_{1C}$) of $\leq 6\%$, and it should be maintained during pregnancy. Macrosomia continues to be a problem, even in well-controlled mothers. Much more on this subject later in this section.

ASSESSING FETAL HEALTH

Fundal Height

Fundal height measurements are still very important and continue to be the simplest screening method to detect IUGR. Remember: The fundal height is taken from the top of the uterine fundus to the symphysis pubis.

Ultrasound Imaging and Biometry

Note: Until 20 weeks, almost all fetuses grow at the same rate! Therefore, it is useful to do an ultrasound at 18–20 weeks to determine gestational age/fetal size. After 20 weeks, fetuses grow at different rates, so measurements will not correlate as well.

The typical fetal ultrasound involves 4 standard measurements:
1) Biparietal diameter of the head
2) Head circumference
3) Abdominal circumference
4) Femur length

Measure these in a "level 1" ultrasound. "Level 2" is much more specialized and helps ascertain if neurologic, heart, GI, GU, and/or skeletal abnormalities exist. If concerns arise during ultrasound, most obstetricians proceed to an amniocentesis for karyotyping.

Nonstress Testing

Nonstress testing (NST) consists of detecting the fetal heart rate (FHR), fetal movement, and uterine activity by external methods, noting the presence of FHR variability with fetal movement. A "reactive" test is 2 accelerations of the FHR in 20 minutes, which is associated with fetal survival of 99% for another week or more. A "nonreactive" test is associated with poor fetal outcome in 20% of cases. Note: The specificity of a "nonreactive" test is not great—80% will be "normal"—so a "nonreactive" test requires further testing,

usually with the "biophysical profile" or a contraction stress test (see below).

Biophysical Profile

The biophysical profile assesses the following 5 factors. The NST determines the first factor; the other 4 are determined by U/S for a maximum of ≤ 30 minutes (if the fetus achieves perfect scores up to that point):
1) Fetal movement
2) Fetal tone
3) Fetal reactivity
4) Fetal breathing
5) Amniotic fluid volume

Points are given, 0–2 for each factor. If the fetus scores a total of ≤ 4 for the combined 5 factors, the obstetrician should consider emergent delivery.

Recently, some obstetricians have been using the "modified biophysical profile," which incorporates the NST and amniotic fluid index (AFI). The modified biophysical profile involves doing an ultrasound and dividing the uterus into 4 parts, with the linea nigra and the umbilicus as dividing points. Scan each quadrant and measure in centimeters the largest pocket of fluid in each quadrant; then total the 4 measurements, with the sum as the AFI. An AFI at 5.1–24 cm is considered normal. An AFI < 5.1 cm is considered oligohydramnios. An AFI of ≥ 24 cm is polyhydramnios.

Contraction Stress Test

This test notes changes in FHR in response to breast stimulation or oxytocin. It requires 3 contractions—each lasting at least 1 minute—recorded over a period of 10 minutes.

Fetal Heart Rate Monitoring

The fetal heart monitor displays 2 components:
1) FHR—usually expressed by the R wave of the fetal electrocardiogram, or via a signal generated by the movement of a part of the fetal heart using ultrasound and Doppler.
2) Uterine contractions—measured by external means using a tocodynamometer, which is placed on the mother's abdomen and recognizes tightening and relaxing of the abdominal musculature during contractions. Uterine contractions can alternately be measured transcervically by use of a catheter inserted into the amniotic cavity and attached to a strain gauge transducer.

If the fetal monitor is attached directly to the fetus (fetal scalp monitor), or directly into the uterine cavity, it is called a "direct," "internal," or "invasive" device. Devices that are not directly in contact with the fetus or the uterine cavity are called "noninvasive" or "external."

ACOG states that intermittent auscultation of the FHR is equivalent to continuous, electronic FHR monitoring if done within specific intervals. This protocol calls for auscultation every 30 minutes for low-risk patients in the active phase of labor, and every 15 minutes in the second stage of labor. Continuous, electronic fetal monitoring is recommended for

notes

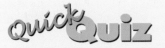

all high-risk patients and, in any case, where abnormalities occur with intermittent auscultation.

Which mothers are considered high risk? (See Table 8-1.)

Note: The validity of fetal monitoring has recently been called into question. The concern is that the false-positive rate for continuous, electronic fetal monitoring is resulting in an unnecessary increase in C-sections and forceps deliveries. (P.S. It has never been shown that fetal monitoring improves ultimate pregnancy outcomes!)

On the Board exam, you are likely to be given an infant with "nonreassuring" patterns on FHR recordings. In such a case, your choice should be to proceed to fetal scalp stimulation, pH measurement, or both. If, on the other hand, the exam question refers to "ominous" patterns, your choice should be to proceed to immediate delivery.

Table 8-2 lists nonreassuring patterns. Table 8-3 lists ominous patterns.

FHR assessment is probably equal, or even superior, to measurement of fetal blood pH in the prediction of good vs. bad outcomes. Fetuses will usually respond with an acceleration of FHR following fetal scalp stimulation; this

tends to correlate with a normal pH; i.e., > 7.25. If fetal scalp stimulation does not induce an increase in FHR, perform fetal scalp sampling for pH. If fetal scalp sampling cannot be done, immediate delivery should proceed based on the lack of response to fetal scalp stimulation.

A scalp pH of 7.20–7.25 is considered "suspicious." Such a measurement should be repeated in 15–30 minutes and also assessed in light of the current FHR pattern and progress of labor. A scalp pH < 7.20 is considered abnormal and generally indicates need for immediate delivery.

Fetal Heart Rate Patterns

The autonomic nervous system controls the FHR. The vagus nerve controls the inhibitory influence, while the sympathetic nervous system controls the excitatory influence. The vagal aspect dominates closer to term and continues after birth, resulting in a gradual decrease in baseline heart rates. Stimulation of the fetus by its own movement or by uterine contractions results in an increase in FHR.

The normal FHR is 120–160 beats/minute (bpm). A "changed" baseline is said to occur if the rate has changed for > 15 minutes.

An example of a "reassuring" pattern would be a baseline heart rate of 130–140 bpm, with preserved, beat-to-beat, and long-term variability. Accelerations may last for ≥ 15 seconds above baseline and peak at ≥ 15 bpm. Clinically, loss of beat-to-beat variability is more significant than loss of long-term variability.

Table 8-1: High-Risk Mothers
Gestational diabetes
Hypertension
Asthma
Multiple gestations
Post-date gestation
Previous C-section
IUGR
PROM
Congenital malformations
Third-trimester bleeding
Oxytocin induction
Preeclampsia
No prenatal care
Tobacco/drug abuse

Table 8-2: Nonreassuring Patterns
Fetal tachycardia
Fetal bradycardia
Saltatory variability
Variable decelerations associated with a nonreassuring pattern
Late decelerations with preserved beat-to-beat variability

Table 8-3: Ominous Patterns
Persistent late decelerations with loss of beat-to-beat variability
Nonreassuring variable decelerations associated with loss of beat-to-beat variability
Prolonged severe bradycardia
Sinusoidal pattern
Confirmed loss of beat-to-beat variability not associated with fetal quiescence, medication, or severe prematurity

notes

Saltatory Pattern: This refers to increased variability in the baseline FHR when the oscillations are > 25 bpm. This is usually caused by acute hypoxia or mechanical compression of the umbilical cord. If seen with late decelerations, this pattern should alert the obstetrician to correct possible causes of acute hypoxia—and to watch for signs that the hypoxia is progressing to acidosis. This is a "nonreassuring" pattern but is usually not an indication for immediate delivery.

Fetal Tachycardia: This is defined by a baseline FHR > 160 bpm. It also is considered a "nonreassuring" pattern. It is "mild" at 160–180 bpm and "severe" when > 180 bpm. Tachycardia > 200 bpm is usually due to a fetal tachyarrhythmia or congenital anomalies and is not due to hypoxia. Persistent tachycardia > 180 bpm that is associated with maternal fever is usually suggestive of chorioamnionitis. The common causes of fetal tachycardia are listed in Table 8-4.

Note: Fetal tachycardia may be a sign of increased fetal stress when it persists for ≥ 10 minutes, but it usually is not associated with severe fetal distress unless decreased variability or another finding is present.

Fetal Bradycardia: This is defined as a baseline heart rate of < 120 bpm. Bradycardia at 100–120 bpm with normal variability is not associated with fetal acidosis. This is pretty common in post-date fetuses and in those fetuses with occiput posterior or transverse presentations. Bradycardia < 100 bpm is seen in fetuses with congenital heart abnormalities or myocardial conduction defects—think systemic lupus erythematosus (SLE)—but bradycardia due to SLE is not usually seen during labor. Bradycardia that is at 80–100 bpm is classified as a nonreassuring pattern. Bradycardia that is ≤ 80 bpm for > 3 minutes is considered ominous, indicates significant hypoxia, and often is associated with death. Table 8-5 lists causes of severe bradycardia, which, unless corrected quickly, can frequently result in fetal death.

Decelerations ("decels"):

Early decels are usually due to fetal head compression during uterine contraction and result in vagal stimulation with slowing of heart rate. This is easy to see on the monitor: The heart rate goes down as the contraction force increases. So you will see a "valley" for the heart rate at the same time you see a "mountain" for the contraction. It gives a mirror image effect on the tracings. These are not associated with fetal distress.

Late decels are a fall in FHR—usually at the beginning, or after the peak, of the uterine contraction—with the return of the FHR only after the contraction has ended. So you'll see the "mountain" peak in the contraction tracing, while the FHR simultaneously starts to fall. The fall in FHR is symmetric, gradual, and smooth. Remember: All late decels are considered potentially ominous. If they are persistent, further evaluate via fetal pH. Late decels are usually seen with uteroplacental insufficiency, which is "unmasked" by uterine contractions.

Variable decels are an acute fall in FHR with a rapid downslope and a variable recovery period. These are commonly encountered patterns during normal labor, but are also seen frequently in women who have experienced PROM and oligohydramnios. They are due to compression of the umbilical cord, which initially occludes the umbilical vein, resulting in an acceleration. Continued pressure will occlude an umbilical artery, resulting in a quick, sharp down-slope in FHR, followed by a quick, sharp up-slope in FHR when the pressure is relieved. Variable decels are generally associated with a favorable outcome. It is mainly a concern if a persistently variable decel pattern develops. Table 8-6 lists signs that a variable decel pattern may be indicative of hypoxia.

Sinusoidal Pattern: This pattern is very rare but if it occurs is very ominous and associated with high morbidity and mortality. It occurs when the FHR shows a sine wave pattern with a frequency of 2–5 cycles/minute and an amplitude of 5–15 bpm. It indicates severe fetal anemia, as seen in Rh disease or severe hypoxia.

Table 8-4: Etiologies of Fetal Tachycardia
Fetal hypoxia
Maternal fever
Hyperthyroidism
Maternal or fetal anemia
Drugs (atropine, hydroxyzine, ritodrine, terbutaline)
Chorioamnionitis
Fetal tachyarrhythmia
Prematurity

Table 8-5: Etiologies of Severe Bradycardia
Prolonged cord compression
Cord prolapse
Tetanic uterine contractions
Paracervical block
Epidural and spinal anesthesia
Maternal seizures
Rapid descent in the birth canal
Vigorous vaginal examination

notes

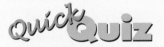

CESAREAN SECTION (C-SECTION)

In the U.S., ~ 25% of babies are delivered via C-section.

The indications for C-section are varied, but generally fall into 5 basic categories:
1) Previous C-section
2) Dystocia
3) "Fetal distress"
4) Malpresentation
5) The generalized "other"

C-section rates have risen dramatically in the past 30 years and vary from community to community, hospital to hospital, and physician to physician. These higher C-section rates have been criticized because of the concomitant rise in morbidity and mortality rates for mothers.

Note: 70% of women with a history of previous C-section (usually with low-transverse cuts) are candidates for a trial vaginal delivery (but see last sentence in this paragraph). Of these, 70% will be successful. Also, ~ 50% of term breeches could successfully be delivered vaginally. Today, there is a lot of controversy about vaginal birth after cesarean (VBACs) because of a report several years ago that told of the increased risk of uterine rupture with attendant neonatal morbidity and mortality.

Table 8-6: Signs That Variable Decelerations May Indicate Fetal Hypoxia
Increased severity of the decel
Late onset and gradual return phase
Blunt acceleration or "overshoot" after severe decel
Unexplained tachycardia
Saltatory variability
Late decels or late return to baseline
Decreased variability

OPERATIVE VAGINAL DELIVERY

Operative vaginal delivery usually is done with forceps or vacuum extraction. Use of forceps has decreased dramatically, with a subsequent increase in vacuum extraction; both are safe if performed with appropriate skill and precautions. The use of forceps has decreased, mainly because of medical-legal repercussions for a comparative minority of bad outcomes and a tendency toward the failure of ob/gyn residents to be taught this method. Indications for operative vaginal delivery are usually related to fetal factors, such as FHR abnormalities or the maternal indicator of prolonged second-stage labor.

The use of either forceps or vacuum is restricted by the amount of force and the number of attempts. The fetal head should descend with each traction attempt. If it fails to do so, the technique should be abandoned. A vacuum may generally be used a maximum of 3 (or, rarely, 4) times. Fetal trauma is usually limited to temporary bruising or skin lacerations.

Anesthesia has changed the length of the second stage of labor. Generally, the second stage is 3 hours for nulliparous women and 2 hours for parous women before operative vaginal delivery should be considered.

Forceps delivery > 0 station is rarely justified or attempted. By definition, +5 is delivered head; +2 to +4 is considered "low;" 0 to +2 station is considered "mid;" and at the pelvic outlet is considered "outlet."

FETAL-TO-NEWBORN TRANSITIONS

Circulatory Transition After Birth

In healthy children, blood circulates from the right side of the heart to the lung, then through the left side of the heart to the systemic circulation before it returns to the right side of the heart. Cardiac output is the volume of blood ejected per minute by either ventricle. In the fetus, this circulation does not occur because the right ventricle ejects only a small amount of blood into the lungs. Most of the right ventricular output passes directly into the systemic circulation through the ductus arteriosus. Fetal cardiac output is the total output of both ventricles and is termed "combined ventricular output," or "CVO." About 40% of the CVO goes to the umbilical-placental circulation.

Blood oxygenated in the placenta returns to the fetus through the umbilical vein. The main umbilical vein passes from the umbilicus to the portal venous system via the porta hepatis. This vein provides the portal branches to the left lobe of the liver and then gives rise to the ductus venosus before it joins the portal vein. The portal veins entering the right lobe of the liver supply a mixture of well-oxygenated, umbilical venous blood and poorly oxygenated, portal venous blood.

The venous supply to the left lobe of the liver is exclusively from the umbilical vein, which is why the left lobe of the liver has a higher oxygen concentration than the right lobe. Accounting for ~ 1/2 of the umbilical venous return, the ductus venosus passes from the umbilical vein directly to the inferior vena cava, and thus bypasses the hepatic circulation completely. The ductus venosus also has a higher oxygenation percentage. The other 1/2 of the umbilical venous return goes through the liver and eventually to the inferior vena cava via the hepatic veins.

Note: Within the vena cava, the blood from the ductus venosus and the left hepatic veins (with their higher oxygenations) do not mix with the blood from the hepatic venous systems, even though they all enter the vena cava! The blood from the ductus venosus and the left hepatic veins enter higher in the inferior vena cava, and get preferentially passed on to the right atrium through the foramen ovale. From there, higher oxygenated blood is provided to the left atrium and left ventricle. The right hepatic blood (which is less oxygenated) enters more distally into the inferior vena cava and passes preferentially to the right atrium and right ventricle (with little going through the foramen ovale).

The fetal brain receives ~ 20–30% of CVO, and the ratio of right-to-left ventricular output is ~ 1.3:1. About 55% of the CVO is ejected by the right ventricle and about 45% by the left.

The oxygen tension of fetal arterial blood is much lower than in the arterial blood of children. Umbilical venous blood flowing through the ductus venosus, or the left hepatic vein, has an oxygen tension of ~ 28–30 mmHg.

Blood in the distal vena cava, superior vena cava, and portal vein has an oxygen tension of about 12–14 mmHg. Left ventricular blood is mainly distributed to the myocardium, brain, and upper body with an oxygen tension of 24–28 mmHg.

Remember: The fetus is surrounded by amniotic fluid, so all fetal pressures are relative to amniotic cavity pressures.
- The vena cava and right atrial pressures are ~ 3–5 mmHg above amniotic cavity pressure.
- Left atrial pressure is 2–4 mmHg above amniotic cavity pressure.
- Right and left ventricular systolic pressures are generally equal, approaching 65–70 mmHg near term.
- Near term, right ventricle, and pulmonary artery pressures are often 5–8 mmHg higher than left ventricle and aorta pressures because of constriction of the ductus arteriosus.

So everything is going along smoothly for the fetus, then the baby is delivered and starts breathing. Now what happens?

The umbilical-placental circulation ceases, and a new pulmonary circulation must start immediately. The umbilical vessels constrict after they are torn or cut, and they also constrict when exposed to higher oxygen tensions.

Once the placental circulation is removed, venous return through the inferior vena cava is markedly reduced. Also, the cessation of umbilical venous return reduces flow through the ductus venosus, which anatomically closes 3–7 days after birth.

Why is the pulmonary blood flow in the fetus so low? Because of high pulmonary vascular resistance. The small arteries in the fetal lungs have a thick, medial, smooth, muscular layer; and they are tonically constricted, resulting in the increased pulmonary vascular resistance. The pulmonary vascular resistance decreases near term as the total cross-sectional area of the lungs expands, due to a large increase in the total number of vessels. Once ventilation and resultant lung expansion occurs, pulmonary vascular resistance markedly decreases, resulting in greatly increased flow through the lungs. This is due to multiple factors, including oxygen itself, prostaglandin release, nitrous oxide, and a host of other factors. Persistence of pulmonary vasoconstriction (persistent pulmonary hypertension of the newborn) may occur in distressed infants as a result of hypothermia, acidosis, hypoxia, and/or hypercapnia.

To review, the changes in pressures and flow:
- Mean pulmonary artery pressure drops dramatically at birth
- Pulmonary blood flow increases dramatically at birth
- Pulmonary vascular resistance drops dramatically at birth

What happens with the foramen ovale?

Remember: In the fetus, 1/2 of the inferior vena cava flow comes from umbilical venous return. Once the placental circulation is cut off, the newborn's circulation gets a marked decrease in the amount of inferior vena cava blood that is returning to the heart. This results in a decrease in right atrial pressure. At the same time, the newborn's circulation is experiencing a huge increase in pulmonary blood flow, which also increases pulmonary venous return. The left atrial pressure rises while the right atrial pressure falls; this results in the foramen ovale closing. Note: A small foramen ovale opening can persist in 15–20% of humans throughout life, but this is not associated with shunting. In some newborns, the foramen ovale can persist with a small, left-to-right shunt for several months.

What happens to the ductus arteriosus?

Note: The ductus in the fetus is about the size of the fetus's descending aorta! We think that, probably, the patency of the ductus, even in utero, is maintained by prostaglandins. The ductus is relaxed by prostacyclin I_2 (PGI_2), and much more importantly, by prostaglandin E_2 (PGE_2). After delivery, the ductus constricts rapidly and is usually "functionally" closed off by 10–15 hours of age. The actual physical closure (i.e., thrombus, fibrosis) doesn't occur for ≥ 3 weeks. Why the ductus closes is still not completely understood. It is likely due to falling levels of PGE_2. Note: While the ductus is still patent immediately after birth, the reduction in pulmonary vascular resistance results in a left-to-right shunt. If pulmonary vascular resistance is increased (frequently due to hypoxia), right-to-left shunting will occur. The ductus likely constricts in the face of the increase in blood oxygen levels that occurs following birth. In an infant with continued

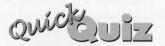

hypoxia after birth, the ductus may remain patent. It is interesting that, in infants born above altitudes of 3,000 feet, there is increased incidence of patent ductus!

Respiratory Transitions

Within minutes after birth, regular breathing is initiated and maintained, lung compliance improves, airway resistance is diminished, and functional residual capacity is established. What is the major factor in this event? Surfactant!—made in the Type II cells that line the distal air spaces. Surfactant lowers surface tension of the alveolar lining layer. If low surface tension does not develop, air spaces collapse near end-expiration. This is what underlies the pathophysiology of respiratory distress in premature infants. For the newborn, it is also very important to clear fluid from the lung air spaces. Most of the fluid is resorbed across the respiratory epithelium, a process driven by transcellular movement of sodium from the lung liquid into the interstitium. Failure to replace pulmonary alveolar fluid with air may lead to signs of respiratory distress (tachypnea, grunting, nasal flaring)—also known as transient tachypnea of the newborn.

Glucose Transitions

In the third trimester, glucose concentrations in the fetus are ~ 80% of maternal levels. Glucose crosses the placenta, and almost all of this is used by the fetus for energy. The fetus does not synthesize its own glucose under normal resting conditions.

So what happens when the umbilical cord is clamped at delivery? Glucose transport to the baby is stopped immediately! Both glycogenolysis and gluconeogenesis maintain glucose production. The serum glucose concentration is maintained at ~ 70 mg/dL. In the neonate, the brain is consuming a large amount of this glucose. Note: Hepatic glycogen stores start to increase significantly only near the end of the third trimester, so a premature infant is at increased risk for hypoglycemia. Use of exogenous glucose is important in these infants, as well as in older infants with signs of hypoglycemia.

Water Balance

At term, infants are 75–80% water, 2/3 of which is intracellular and 1/3 extracellular. During the first week of life, water loss accounts for a large percentage of the body's weight loss. Most of this water loss is intracellular and interstitial. Premature babies will lose an increased amount of body water early on.

THE DELIVERY ROOM

APGAR

Dr. Virginia Apgar designed an important scoring system to help assess an infant's physiological status soon after birth. See Table 8-7 for the actual system. The Apgar score at 1 and 5 minutes after birth does not correlate well with long-term, neurobehavioral results; but a score of < 3 at 15 minutes has been associated with > 50% mortality and > 60% permanent, severe neurologic sequelae in infants who survive. Sometimes on the Boards, you'll be given various findings in the Apgar scoring system and asked to provide the corresponding Apgar score.

DELIVERY ROOM RESUSCITATION

Overview

Administer oxygen via free-flowing system if the infant is cyanotic and has a heart rate > 100 beats/minute (or if the infant has a measured pulse oximeter reading < 85%). If the infant's heart rate is < 100 bpm, or the infant appears to be unable to breathe normally, initiate positive pressure ventila-

Table 8-7: Apgar Scores			
SCORE	0	1	2
Heart rate	Absent	< 100 beats/min	> 100 beats/min
Respiration	Absent	Slow, irregular	Good, crying
Muscle tone	Limp	Some flexion	Active motion
Reflex irritability*	No response	Grimace	Cough, sneeze, cry
Color	Blue, pale	Body pink, blue limbs	Completely pink

*Reflex irritability is tested in response to a catheter placed in the infant's nose.
Scoring is done at 1 minute, 5 minutes.
Maximum score is 10.

notes

tion. It is important to remember not to over-oxygenate! Studies show that hyperoxemia will result in damage. It is best to keep the PaO_2 at 50–70 mmHg and the oxygen saturation at 90–95%.

If apnea develops or breathing is not adequate, begin assisted ventilation. You usually can start this in the delivery room with a bag-and-mask device. Inflation pressures of 25 cm H_2O at rates of 25–40 breaths/min are normally adequate. If this is not effective, insert an endotracheal tube. The size (i.e., diameter) of the endotracheal tube is important, and you must estimate this size in the delivery room, based on weight:

< 1.5 kg wt.—2.5 mm tube dia.
1.5–2.5 kg wt. —3 mm tube dia.
> 2.5 kg wt.—3.5 mm tube dia.

Length of tubes, measured from the distal end to the baby's lips, is similarly based on weight:

1 kg wt.—7 cm tube length
2 kg wt.—8 cm tube length
3 kg wt.—9 cm tube length
4 kg wt.—10 cm tube length

These lengths should place the distal end of the endotracheal tube 1 cm above the bifurcation of the trachea.

What about the heart? If it is beating < 60 bpm and this continues even after adequate ventilation, initiate external cardiac compressions: For newborns, use both thumbs on the lower third of the sternum and gently surround the chest with the fingers of both hands to support the back. Compress the sternum 1/3 the depth of the anterior-posterior diameter of the chest. The compressions should be in a 3:1 ratio of compressions to ventilations with 90 compressions and 30 breaths to achieve approximately 120 events/minute. Thus, each event takes 1/2 second, with exhalation occurring during the 1st compression after each ventilation.

Cardiac Arrest: Initiate positive pressure ventilation and external cardiac compressions. If there is no response, drugs may need to be administered. Epinephrine is most commonly given first.

Epinephrine [Know!]:
• Stimulates α-adrenergic receptors
• Enhances cardiac contractility
• Constricts the peripheral circulation
• Has β-adrenergic effects on the receptors in the heart
• Increases rate and effectiveness of cardiac contraction

The dose is 0.01–0.03 mg/kg of 1:10,000 solution IV (preferred) or endotracheal. The most common cause of bradycardia in an infant is ineffective bag-mask ventilation, esophageal intubation, or airway obstruction. An arrhythmia-like ventricular fibrillation is rare in cardiac arrests in newborns; but if it occurs, administer 2 Joules/kg to the infant's chest.

Drugs

Condition of the newborn determines the use of drugs, if any. The peripheral or umbilical vein is the customary site for intravascular access, but you must be certain of its location before administering hyperosmolar solutions. Situate the tip of an umbilical venous catheter in the inferior vena cava above the diaphragm to reduce the risk of liver damage via direct instillation into the portal vein. An alternative would be to insert an umbilical vein catheter just until blood flow is obtained, generally 2–3 cm past the abdominal ring.

Remember: Epinephrine and atropine may be given via endotracheal tube. (But, the IV route is preferred.)

Sodium bicarbonate ($NaHCO_3$): Indicated if severe metabolic acidosis is present. The initial dose is 2 mEq/kg and should be administered no faster than 0.5–1 mEq/kg/minute. The concern with $NaHCO_3$ administration is that it increases $PaCO_2$, so ensure that adequate ventilation is in place. If the $PaCO_2$ remains elevated, use tromethamine (THAM) instead of $NaHCO_3$, because it will bind CO_2 in addition to H+ ions.

Calcium gluconate/chloride: Rarely used in neonatal resuscitation.

Glucose: Hypoglycemia may occur during resuscitation. If this happens, infuse 10% solution of IV glucose at a rate of 2–3 mL/kg, with a continuous infusion thereafter.

Naloxone (Narcan®): Give if the mother is suspected of using, or has been administered, narcotics. But, avoid if the mother has known long-term use of opioids because of the risk of precipitating acute withdrawal in infants who have chronically been exposed to narcotics. Use 0.1 mg/kg IM or IV, and repeat as necessary. Also be aware that naloxone has a half-life of 2–3 hours, which can be shorter than some of the longer-lived narcotics used for maternal anesthesia.

Dopamine: Useful if the infant has experienced cardiomyopathy and/or hypotension. The usual dose is 5–10 µg/kg/min.

Blood volume expanders: Useful when hypotension is present, and it is thought to be due to intravascular volume loss. The condition can manifest in several ways—tachycardia, metabolic acidosis, poor peripheral perfusion, and/or severe pallor. If you believe blood loss is the etiology, it is best to replace intravascular volume with whole blood or packed RBCs. If blood is not available immediately, use isotonic saline.

Antibiotics may be indicated if sepsis is a suspected etiology. These are discussed in the Infectious Disease section.

THE NEWBORN EXAMINATION
OVERVIEW

Proper examination of a newborn is ongoing throughout the hospital stay. Every time you interact with the infant, you should be making observations. For example, how well does he/she feed? What's the quality and content of maternal interactions? Is diapering being handled appropriately? Your first formal newborn examination should be conducted within 24 hours after birth.

notes

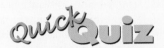

Quick Quiz

1) What is the best value to keep the PaO$_2$ in the newborn?

2) Know which size endotracheal tube to use, based on birth weight.

3) What does epinephrine do to the heart in a "code" situation?

4) What is the dose of epinephrine for neonates?

5) What 2 neonatal resuscitation drugs can be given via the endotracheal tube?

6) What drug, and at what dose, can you give if you suspect the child is sedated due to maternal anesthetics or narcotics?

7) At what gestational age would you expect to find vernix just on the back, scalp, and creases?

8) At what gestational age would you expect to find an ear with the upper 2/3 incurving?

9) At what gestational age would you expect to find only 1 or 2 anterior creases on the soles?

10) At what gestational age would you expect to find nails that extend well past the fingertips?

11) At what gestational age would you expect to find lanugo on the shoulders only?

GESTATIONAL AGE / SIZE

There are several methods to assess gestational age:
- Number of days since the first day of the last menstrual cycle (if known and the mother's menstrual cycle has been regular/consistent)
- Dates determined by U/S taken at 18–20 weeks gestation
- Use of physical characteristics of the newborn (see below)

Following are points the ABP exam will likely ask you. It is a pain to remember these, but know them!

Vernix:
- Covers body in a thick layer: 24–38 weeks
- Just on back, scalp, creases: 38–39 weeks
- In the creases and scant: 40–41 weeks
- No vernix: > 42 weeks

Breast tissue and areola:
- Areola and nipple barely visible; no breast tissue: 24–33 weeks
- Areola raised: 34–35 weeks
- Breast tissue a 1–2 mm nodule: 36–37 weeks
- Breast tissue a 3–5 mm nodule: 38 weeks
- Breast tissue a 5–6 mm nodule: 39 weeks
- Breast tissue a 7–10 mm nodule: ≥ 40 weeks

Ear:
Form:
- Flat, shapeless: 24–33 weeks
- Superior incurving beginning: 34–35 weeks
- Upper 2/3 incurving: 36–38 weeks
- Well-defined incurving to lobe: ≥ 39 weeks

Cartilage:
- Pinna soft, stays folded: 24–31 weeks
- Cartilage scant, returns slowly from folding: 32–35 weeks
- Thin cartilage, springs back from folding: 36–39 weeks
- Pinna firm, remains erect from head: ≥ 40 weeks

Sole creases:
- No anterior sole creases: 24–31 weeks
- 1–2 anterior creases: 32–33 weeks
- 2–3 anterior creases: 34–35 weeks
- 2/3 of the anterior sole with creases: 36–37 weeks
- Heel creases present: 38–41 weeks
- Deeper creases over entire sole: ≥ 42 weeks

Skin:
Thickness and appearance:
- Thin, see-through venules on abdomen, edema: 24–31 weeks
- Smooth, thicker, without edema: 32–35 weeks
- Pink: 36–37 weeks
- Few vessels seen: 38–39 weeks
- Desquamation starting; pale pink: 40–41 weeks
- Thick, pale, desquamating over all areas: ≥ 42 weeks

Nail plates:
- Appear at 20–22 weeks
- Nails to finger tips: 32–41 weeks
- Nails extend well beyond fingertips: ≥ 42 weeks

Hair:
- Appears on head: 20–22 weeks
- Eyebrows and eyelashes: 23–27 weeks
- Fine, "woolly," out from head: 28–36 weeks
- Silky, single strands, lies flat: 37–41 weeks
- Receding hairline/loss of baby hair: ≥ 42 weeks

Lanugo:
- Covers entire body: 22–32 weeks
- Disappears from face: 33–37 weeks
- Present on shoulders only: 38–41 weeks
- None present: ≥ 42 weeks

Genitals:
Testes:
- Palpable in inguinal canal: 28–35 weeks
- Palpable in upper scrotum: 36–39 weeks
- Palpable in lower scrotum: ≥ 40 weeks

notes

Scrotum:
- Few rugae: 28–35 weeks
- Rugae especially on anterior portion: 36–39 weeks
- Rugae cover the entire scrotum: 40–41 weeks
- "Pendulous": ≥ 42 weeks

Labia and clitoris:
- Prominent clitoris; labia majora small and separate: 30–35 weeks
- Labia majora almost covers clitoris: 36–39 weeks
- Labia minora and clitoris covered: ≥ 40 weeks

Skull firmness:
- Bones are soft: up to 27 weeks
- Soft to 1 inch from anterior fontanelle: 28–34 weeks
- Spongy at edges of fontanelle with firm center: 35–37 weeks
- Bones hard with sutures movable: 38–41 weeks
- Bones hard, sutures cannot be moved: ≥ 42 weeks

Sanity Break

OK, that's a lot of stuff to remember, but go creative instead of crazy. Remember: Most of us did this daily when we did our "newborn nursery" rotation and deliveries. For many of you that's a long time ago, but just take it slow and concentrate on the subjects the Boards really like to ask about: lanugo, genitals, soles, breast buds, and ears. The exam asks about the others too, but if you can at least get those 5 down cold, you'll go a long way toward bettering your odds for the Boards!

Back to Work

Now back to the physical examination of the newborn. Always measure the birth weight, head circumference, and crown-to-heel length. Once you have these measurements and the gestational age, you can plot them on growth charts. Measurements are appropriate for gestational age (AGA) if they fall within ± 2 standard deviations of "normal." With regard to birth weight, an infant < the 10th percentile is small for gestational age (SGA), and an infant > the 90th percentile is large for gestational age (LGA). Remember also: Some infants are disproportionate with regard to head circumference, length, or weight. Depending on what is "out of whack," they can be at increased risk for neurologic abnormalities (head circumference) or hypoglycemia (weight).

CRYING IN THE NEWBORN

During the first few hours of life, the baby generally will spend 80% of the time sleeping. The remaining awake time is spent with or without crying. It is very important to pay attention to the cry of the infant! A weak/whimpering cry or a high-pitched/shrieking cry is abnormal. The latter, in particular, suggests neurologic problems. A hoarse cry suggests vocal cord paralysis, hypothyroidism, or trauma to the hypopharynx. Remember also that infants are obligate nasal breathers—an infant who is cyanotic except when crying likely has bilateral choanal atresia. Confirm by attempting to pass a small feeding tube through the nares into the hypopharynx.

TEMPERATURE

Normal axillary temperature is 36.5–37.4° C. Infants are very susceptible to environmental temperature changes, from being too cool to becoming overheated under a "warmer." Any persistent change in temperature in a normal-temperature environment warrants quick assessment. Sepsis is the biggest concern and can present with fever, hypothermia, or a fluctuating temperature. Also, with hypothermia, look for hypoglycemia, hypothyroidism, or hypoxia. With hyper-thermia, look for drug withdrawal, intracranial hemorrhage, or adrenal hemorrhage.

SKIN

Review the specifications and norms listed above for the lanugo, vernix, skin, and nails. These are commonly asked about on the Boards. Note: If hypoxia occurs *in utero*, meconium may be passed into the amnionic fluid. This will stain the skin, nails, and umbilical cord with a greenish hue if it has been in contact with these areas for several hours.

Blistering skin may be caused by epidermolysis bullosa, but also watch out for staphylococcal infection because this infection will need emergent treatment! But don't confuse blistering with peeling skin in a neonate after a post-date pregnancy.

Aplasia cutis: A congenital absence of skin that usually occurs just in a small, localized area (see Figure 8-2). If it occurs in multiple places on the top of the scalp, look for trisomy 13! If it occurs as a midline defect, look for spinal dysraphia!

Color: Changes in skin color can be helpful in determining certain abnormalities.

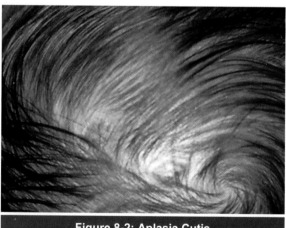
Figure 8-2: Aplasia Cutis

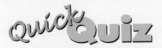

Here are some examples:

- Pallor: Anemia or poor perfusion.
- Pale, mottled skin: Sepsis or hypothermia.
- Acrocyanosis: Cyanosis of the hands and feet if exposed to colder temperatures—this can be a normal finding.
- Generalized cyanosis: Methemoglobinemia or significant hypoxemia.
- Plethora: Polycythemia.
- Harlequin skin: This is weird, but it has no pathologic basis. Likely the result of vasomotor instability, one side of the baby will be pink while the other side turns pale, with a sharp line of demarcation in the midline. (See Figure 8-3.)
- Ecchymoses: Usually due to birth trauma and without significance. Severe trauma, however, can result in bleeding into the underlying muscle with hemorrhage.
- Petechiae: Scattered, localized petechiae common after delivery, especially of the presenting part. Extensive petechiae should lead to greater concern about thrombocytopenia.
- Subcutaneous fat necrosis: Most commonly occurs on the cheeks, buttocks, limbs, and back—exhibited by an overlaying redness on the skin, which is rubbery and firm on palpation. Not usually a problem. A rare complication is hypercalcemia, presenting at 1–6 months of age with

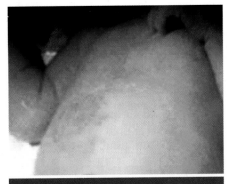

Figure 8-3: Harlequin Skin

lethargy, poor feeding, and failure to thrive. The origin of the hypercalcemia is unclear—cardiac, central nervous system, and renal complications may occur.

- Jaundice: If present the first day, it warrants immediate evaluation—be most concerned about sepsis or hemolytic anemia! It is fairly normal for neonatal jaundice to occur during days 2–4 of life, with an increase in indirect reacting bilirubin. More on jaundice later.

Rashes are very common in the newborn. They are reviewed in the Dermatology and Infectious Disease sections.

THE HEAD

Shape

Head shape will vary depending on the birth position—vertex, breech, or C-section. With vertex delivery, there can be vertical elongation of the head. Breech babies will have a prominent occipital shelf.

Always palpate the sutures; they should be palpably open and can be separated up to a few millimeters. Molding is temporary overlapping of the bones and must be distinguished from craniosynostosis (premature closure of the sutures).

Fontanelles

The anterior fontanelle is open, soft, and flat at birth, and its mean diameter is < 3.5 cm. The posterior fontanelle is often only fingertip size, or just barely open. Any bulging or tense fontanelle indicates increased intracranial pressure and requires immediate workup. A large fontanelle may be associated with hydrocephalus, hypothyroidism, and rickets. The combination of persistent posterior fontanelle, umbilical hernia, and jaundice is hypothyroidism! Craniotabes, soft areas away from the fontanelle, have a "ping-pong ball" feel and are the result of in utero compression. Craniotabes are also associated with hydrocephalus, rickets, and syphilis.

Craniosynostosis

Some form of craniosynostosis may occur once in every 2,000 births. The specific pathophysiology is not understood. We know that the skull grows perpendicular to the suture lines. For example, premature closure of the sagittal suture prevents growth in the coronal direction, resulting in a long, thin head (scaphocephaly). The shape of the head in craniosynostosis is a function of which suture has prematurely closed.

Sagittal: long, thin head shape causing scaphocephaly (see Figure 8-4)

Coronal: broad, short, anterior-posterior dimension causing brachycephaly (see Figure 8-5)

Lambdoid or single coronal: trapezoidal or parallelogram shape causing plagiocephaly (see Figure 8-6. Although the head appears to be turned to the right, visualize it correctly by imagining the nose on top like the other pictures!)

notes

Metopic: keel-shaped forehead causing trigonocephaly (see Figure 8-7)

Craniosynostosis can be isolated or, if multiple sutures are involved, is likely associated with other syndromes (e.g., Apert syndrome or Crouzon's). Neurologic complications of isolated craniosynostosis are rare. Plain x-rays and CT scans can provide diagnostic information. The earliest sign is increased bone density along the suture.

Treatment is usually cosmetic, unless there is optic nerve compromise or increased intracranial pressure. Surgery is generally a linear craniectomy (removing the fused suture) and is most effective within the first 12 months.

Caput Succedaneum

This is a collection of edema fluid and blood in the soft tissue of the skull, which accumulates over the presenting part and is due to the forces of labor. The incidence is increased with prolonged labor and vacuum extraction. (See Figure 8-8.)

The key is that the edema, which is sometimes ecchymotic, will commonly cross suture lines and the midline of the skull. It is non-pitting in character. The "caput" is external to the periosteum, which allows the edema to spread.

Significant bleeding is rare, but neonatal jaundice can be aggravated because the blood is resorbed.

Skull x-rays are not indicated. The caput will resolve over several days. Remember this one by thinking of a "cap" (as in caput) on top of the head, but not under the periosteum.

Cephalohematoma

This is a collection of blood under the periosteum of the outer surface of the skull. It is due to rupture of blood vessels that run between the skull and periosteum. It occurs in ~ 2.5% of live births. Most commonly, it occurs over the parietal bones. Remember: Since the blood is below the periosteum, it will not cross the suture lines. An "edge" is usually palpable on the mar-

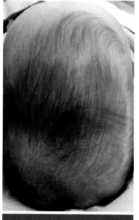

Figure 8-4: Scaphocephaly

gins of the lesion. Of note: Linear skull fractures are found in a minority of newborns with cephalohematomas. Cephalohematomas are not discolored and will usually enlarge during the first few days of life, then slowly resolve over weeks or months. Significant bleeding is a risk. When the blood is resorbed, it can aggravate neonatal jaundice. Aspiration and x-rays are not routinely indicated. Skull fractures, if present, are usually linear and don't require specific therapy. Occasionally, cephalohematoma will calcify but even those lesions are generally self-limited. Infection is rare.

Occipital cephalohematomas are uncommon, but you have to be careful not to confuse them with encephaloceles. The latter will transilluminate, are pulsatile, and are associated with an underlying bony defect. If you can't tell, get a U/S or CT scan.

Subgaleal Hemorrhage

This results from bleeding, occasionally significantly, beneath the scalp aponeurotica. The baby will present with firm, fluctuant swelling over the scalp that extends posteriorly to the neck or in front of the ears. The ears may be pushed out laterally. Infants are at risk of hypotension and/or a consumptive coagulopathy due to massive loss of blood. Hemophilia may present with a subgaleal hemorrhage.

Skull Fractures

Linear: Uncommon, but can occur during an uncomplicated vaginal delivery, as well as during delivery with forceps. Do not do skull x-ray after a "difficult" delivery unless there is evidence of significant head injury—in which case, a CT is likely the better test anyway. Linear skull fractures are benign and have excellent prognosis; but if one is found, quickly look for further trauma. Do follow-up x-rays at 2–3 months to document healing, as well as to exclude development of a leptomeningeal cyst.

Depressed: Associated with forceps but can also occur with spontaneous vaginal delivery. Most are "ping-pong ball" variety and are not associated with loss of bony continuity. Infants usually are neurologically normal and present with just a depressed deformity in their skull. However, bone fragments, hemorrhage, or pressure from the depression can

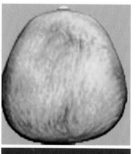

Figure 8-5: Brachycephaly

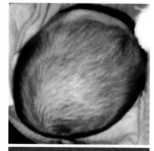

Figure 8-6: Plagiocephaly

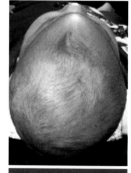

Figure 8-7: Trigonocephaly

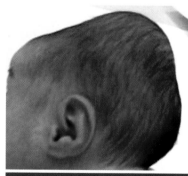

Figure 8-8: Caput Succedaneum

notes

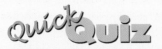

1) True or False: Neurologic complications of isolated craniosynostosis are common.

2) Differentiate caput succedaneum from a cephalohematoma. Which will cross suture lines?

3) How will subgaleal hemorrhage present?

4) Differentiate between linear, depressed, and basal skull fractures.

5) Differentiate between subarachnoid and epidural hemorrhages.

6) What should you think of when you see a "white pupillary reflex"?

7) What eye findings are seen with Horner syndrome?

8) What causes inclusion blennorrhea?

9) How are preauricular pits inherited?

cause damage to the underlying brain. Prognosis is good if neurologic abnormalities are not present.

Basal: Result from occipital bone separation that leads to direct brain injury and disruption of venous structures, with significant bleeding. The bleeding occurs in the posterior fossa and can cause significant morbidity. Overall, prognosis is not good, with a significant risk of permanent sequelae.

Intracranial Bleeding

Subarachnoid hemorrhage: Can occur from birth trauma or hypoxia. Minor hemorrhage is common, but more extensive bleeding can present with seizures. Lumbar puncture or CT scan can diagnose it.

Epidural hemorrhage: Due to bleeding between the bone and periosteum of the inner surface of the skull. It can be arterial or venous. It is rare in the newborn and, if present, is associated with traumatic delivery. It may present with a cephalohematoma or linear skull fracture. Diagnose by CT scan. Surgical evacuation is frequently required, with a guarded prognosis.

Subdural hemorrhage: Usually due to excessive forces of compression of the fetal skull, leading to injury of underlying venous structures. Bleeding from the superficial cerebral veins is pretty common, and may not be associated with abnormalities in the newborn. However, this may present later with macrocephaly, seizures, and developmental delay. If injury occurs to larger cerebral veins, a more acute onset is likely. Diagnosis can be made with CT or MRI. Subdural

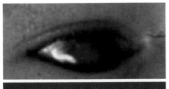

Figure 8-9: Cataract

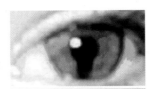

Figure 8-10: Coloboma

effusions can present later in infancy and still be due to birth trauma, but also investigate the possibility of child abuse.

EYES

The ophthalmoscopic examination: Look for cataracts (see Figure 8-9) and colobomas (see Figure 8-10) of the iris. These can appear alone but frequently indicate syndromic involvement. Also, look for red reflex and focus down into the retina to see the vessels. If you see a "white pupillary reflex" (leukokoria), this is abnormal. Think of retinoblastoma, retinal coloboma, chorioretinitis, or retinopathy of prematurity. A cataract will look like a black opacity that interferes with visualization of the lens.

Other basics of eye examination and findings to look for:
An infant should be able to fix and follow at least part of the way while being examined.

Lids: Congenital lid ptosis will show up as "drooping lids." Facial paralysis may present with inability to close the lids completely. Horner syndrome, due to lower brachial plexus injury, which includes the first thoracic nerve, will present with ptosis, miosis, and enophthalmos.

Congenital microphthalmia: It is frequently seen with genetic abnormalities and may be autosomal dominant (AD) or autosomal recessive (AR), depending on the familial trait/abnormality.

Proptosis: If present, look for mass lesions or retrobulbar hemorrhage.

Hemorrhages: Subconjunctival, anterior chamber, vitreous, or retinal hemorrhages may all be seen with birth trauma.

Congenital glaucoma: This appears as an enlarged cornea that becomes progressively cloudy. A corneal diameter of ≥ 11 mm warrants further investigation.

Conjunctivitis: It is usually apparent after the second day of life. Think of bacterial pathogens, especially *Neisseria gonorrhea*, *Staphylococcus aureus*, streptococci, and Gram negatives. The gonococcus is quite serious and can spread rapidly, with panophthalmitis and eye destruction. Gram stain and cultures are recommended before systemic therapy.

Inclusion blennorrhea: This is due to *Chlamydia trachomatis* and appears during the first week of life.

EARS

Examine the ears to be sure they are well formed and contain appropriate cartilage. Things that you may see:

Preauricular pits: Common and AD.

Preauricular skin appendages: Also common.

(Either of these may be associated with deafness if there is a hereditary link.)

Malformed auricles or low-set ears are associated with many syndromes. In particular, be on the lookout for urogenital malformations!

A dull-gray tympanic membrane may be visualized unless the canal is obstructed by vernix.

NOSE

Most newborns are nose-breathers. Unilateral or bilateral anatomic obstruction from choanal atresia is rare. Nasal stuffiness can occur as a result of trauma or because of mucus that is still in the nostrils. Note: Nasal stuffiness can also be a sign of drug withdrawal.

MOUTH

Remember: Examine the mouth by visual inspection, as well as palpation. Even unseen complete or submucosal cleft palates can be palpated. If you see a cleft uvula, also look for a palate defect!

Other things to look for:

Epithelial Pearls: Are common and shiny, white masses (retention cysts) on the gums.

Epstein Pearls: An accumulation of epithelial cells found in the midline, on the roof of the mouth, and at the junction of the hard and soft palates. (See Figure 8-11.)

Ranula: A benign mass that comes out of the floor of the mouth; it is a sublingual dilatation of a salivary gland. It should be excised and the severed duct exteriorized. See Figure 8-12 for an example of one in a youth.

High-arched Palate: Think dysmorphic syndromes.

Narrow Palate: Think dysmorphic syndromes.

Protruding Tongue: Think hemangioma, isolated macroglossia, hypothyroidism, Down syndrome, or Beckwith-Wiedemann syndrome (associated with macrosomia, ear fissures, facial hemangioma, mental retardation, and the big tongue).

A short frenulum (ankyloglossia) should not be surgically cut unless there is difficulty feeding.

Protruding tongue with a small mouth +/– cleft palate: If presented on the Board exam, this will generally be Pierre Robin syndrome!

Natal Teeth: If these occur, they are usually in the lower incisor position (see Figure 8-13). They can be either supernumerary or "true milk" teeth. You can remove supernumerary teeth without problems; however, if they are "true milk" teeth, their removal will leave a hole until the permanent teeth start to erupt in later childhood. This could cause problems for positioning of the molars and dental arch. Rule of thumb: If anything more than a simple pinch is required to remove the tooth, leave it in!

NECK

Cervical Masses: These could be goiters, cavernous hemangioma, or cystic hygroma. Be mindful of tracheal compromise with any of these.

Brachial Cleft Abnormalities: Cysts or sinuses that occur along the anterior margin of the sternocleidomastoid muscle due to improper closure during embryonic life.

Thyroglossal Duct Cysts: Occur in the ventral midline and move vertically with swallowing and tongue protrusion.

Torticollis: Occurs when one of the sternocleidomastoid muscles tightens and the other is absent or atretic, resulting in severe head tilt; also, this is frequently associated with facial abnormalities. A hematoma within the sternocleidomastoid muscle may follow a traumatic delivery and cause torticollis, as can fibrosis caused by fixed positioning *in utero*. Torticollis is also associated with Arnold-Chiari malformation and cervical spine lesions.

Edema and webbing of the neck suggest Turner syndrome.

Erb Paralysis: May occur when there is significant lateral traction during delivery, resulting in damage to the upper part of the brachial plexus—particularly the 5th and 6th cervical roots. This will result in paralysis of the shoulder and arm. The arm will be held alongside the body in internal rotation (known as the "waiter's tip" position—see Figure 8-14). Luckily, this resolves spontaneously in most infants. If not, prescribe physical therapy after the 2nd week. Surgery may be required for recalcitrant cases. Palpate for ipsilateral clavicle fractures!

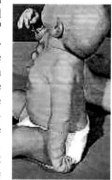

Figure 8-14: Erb Paralysis

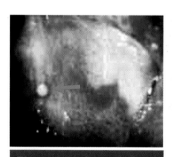

Figure 8-11: Epstein Pearl

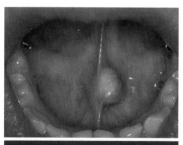

Figure 8-12: Ranula

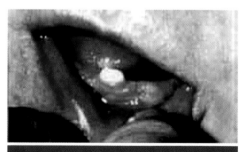

Figure 8-13: Natal Teeth

notes

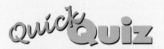
Klumpke Paralysis: Occurs when the lower part of the brachial plexus is damaged. Generally, this will involve the 8th cervical and the 1st thoracic component of the brachial plexus, resulting in a claw-like posturing of the hand. This is most commonly seen with breech deliveries. These are less likely to improve spontaneously than Erb, but still may respond to physical therapy.

Horner Syndrome: Remember—this presents with ptosis, miosis, enophthalmos, and delayed pigmentation of the iris and is caused by injury to the sympathetic fibers of T1.

CHEST

Fracture of the clavicles is the most common injury to the chest. It is usually found by crepitation over the clavicles.

Supernumerary nipples are fairly common, and considered a minor anomaly. Widely spaced nipples with a shield-like chest are seen in Turner syndrome.

Breast hypertrophy is common; milk may be present but should not be expressed. The engorgement may increase during the first few days, but then usually resolves.

LUNGS

Normally, the respiratory rate is 30–40 breaths/minute but can be as high as 60 breaths/minute. A rate consistently > 60 breaths/minute usually indicates a problem—pulmonary, cardiac, or metabolic. With normal breathing, the chest and abdomen move together.

Thoracoabdominal Asynchrony: Occurs when the airway is obstructed or the lungs are stiff. The abdomen will enlarge while the chest cavity gets smaller with inspiration.

Retractions: Evidenced when the tissues between the ribs are sucked in during inspiration. These are normal during the first few minutes after birth; but if they occur later, may indicate stiff lungs or airway obstruction.

Grunting, Nasal flaring, and Tachypnea: Common in the first few minutes after delivery, but their persistence (or later appearance) frequently indicates a respiratory or cardiac abnormality.

Chest Wall Movement: One side of chest moving less than the other indicates an elevated paralyzed diaphragm. Phrenic nerve palsy or an intrathoracic mass can cause this. An example of the intrathoracic mass is a diaphragmatic hernia—almost always on the left, it is associated with bowel sounds in the chest, scaphoid abdomen, and displaced point of maximal cardiac impulse. Note: Phrenic nerve palsy and diaphragmatic hernia can occur without evidence of a paralyzed diaphragm—so be careful to still think of these 2 possibilities in the child with respiratory distress and no evidence of paralyzed diaphragm!

Breath Sounds: Are usually bronchovesicular in the newborn. However, note: Breath sounds may be heard even in a pneumothorax! (Boards: a post-term baby with a history of meconium stained amniotic fluid presenting with respiratory distress may have a pneumothorax due to a meconium plug!)

Coughing: Indicates a serious abnormality in the newborn. Suspect viral pneumonia!

HEART

By palpation, the point of maximal cardiac impulse (PMI) is along the left side of the sternum at the 4th–5th interspace, and usually just medial to the mid-clavicular line. If the PMI is displaced, suspect pneumothorax, dextrocardia, or a space-occupying lesion.

Heart rates generally are 160–180 bpm in the first few hours of life, slowing to 120–130 bpm in the healthy, awake newborn. During sleep, the heart rate may fall to 80 bpm and, on rare occasions, to 60 bpm. A sustained heart rate of < 80 should raise concern. Causes of bradycardia include birth asphyxia, increased intracranial pressure, hypothyroidism, congenital heart disease, and heart block. (Think maternal SLE in an infant with complete heart block!) Tachycardias with sustained rates > 180 bpm should raise concerns of fever, hypovolemia, drug withdrawal, congenital heart disease, tachyarrhythmias, anemia, and hyperthyroidism.

Heart sounds: Murmurs are quite common; only about 8% of murmurs heard at birth indicate significant congenital heart disease. These "benign" murmurs are usually due to transient changes in postnatal circulation.

However, investigate any murmur that is accompanied by:
• cyanosis,
• evidence of poor perfusion,
• tachypnea, or
• that persists after the first day of life.

notes

Systolic blood pressure in term infants < 12 hours of age is usually 60–90 mmHg, with the average ~ 75. Remember: Palpate pulses in all 4 extremities to evaluate for coarctation of the aorta.

ABDOMEN

In the newborn, the liver is normally palpated 1–2 cm below the right costal margin, and the spleen is palpated at no more than 1 cm below the left costal margin. Each kidney is usually palpable, with the right normally lower than the left. The amount you can palpate is usually ~ 2 cm. If more than that is palpable, suspect hydronephrosis, cystic lesions, neoplasm, or renal vein thrombosis.

Abdominal masses, if present, commonly arise from the GU system (hydronephrosis, polycystic kidney disease). Less common origins include the GI system and neoplasms. Trauma during delivery can result in abdominal masses—particularly subcapsular hematomas of the liver. These will present with an elevated diaphragm and, if they rupture, could cause the baby to go into shock. Other trauma-induced abnormalities include adrenal hemorrhage (mass above the kidney, with fever) and splenic rupture.

Abnormalities of the abdominal wall are fairly common and usually benign. Examples:

Diastasis Recti: A midline gap between the abdominal rectus muscles. It is most noticeable with crying. Usually, this will close after the first year of life. Umbilical hernias are also common and are small defects in the periumbilical musculature of the anterior abdominal wall.

Omphalocele: Occurs when abdominal contents pass through a periumbilical defect near the umbilical cord. It can be quite extensive and include the liver, spleen, and intestines, resulting in a mass outside of the body, covered with a membrane that encloses the viscera. (See Figure 8-15.)

Gastroschisis: A defect due to primary failure of the lateral ventral folds, resulting in the small and large intestine sitting outside the abdomen. Unlike an omphalocele, this defect is not covered by a membrane. (See Figure 8-16.)

Prune Belly: Occurs if there is absence of anterior abdominal wall musculature. This is associated with urinary tract anomalies and cryptorchidism.

Single-artery Umbilical Cord: Usually, the umbilical cord has 2 arteries and 1 vein. 1% of newborns will have a single artery, and 15% of these infants will have at least 1 other

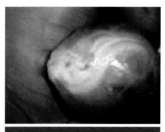

Figure 8-15: Omphalocele

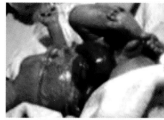

Figure 8-16: Gastroschisis

abnormality. Looking at it differently, 85% of newborns with a single umbilical artery are healthy. The incidence of a single umbilical artery is higher in a multiple pregnancy, with advanced maternal age, and in maternal diabetes mellitus.

Persistent Vitelline Duct: Can persist and may communicate with the umbilicus, with visible umbilical mucus drainage. If it persists, it may create a fistula between the ileum and the umbilicus, and meconium may pass through the umbilicus! If the urachus persists, a fistula tract from the bladder to the umbilicus can result, with urine excretion from the umbilicus.

Delayed Umbilical Cord Separation: Typically, the umbilical cord will fall off within 10–14 days, but it can be normal to take ≥ 3 weeks. Delayed separation of the umbilical cord can occur in infants with defective phagocyte function (leukocyte adhesion deficiency, chronic granulomatous disease).

Umbilical Polyp: A small granuloma that occurs at the site of cord separation. Some mild redness is normal during the first week, but if it becomes more extensive, or deeper in color, suspect omphalitis. This is a serious condition whereby the infection could spread along the umbilical vein to the portal venous sinus of the liver. Most omphalitis cases are polymicrobial in origin; common causative organisms include *Staphylococcus aureus,* group A streptococcus, *Escherichia coli*, *Klebsiella pneumoniae*, and *Proteus mirabilis*. Ectopic GI tissue has been known to masquerade as an umbilical granuloma.

GENITALIA

Females: In term girls, the labia majora meet in the midline, which covers the rest of the genitalia. The urethra is just below the clitoris and must be differentiated from the vagina. A single orifice is obviously abnormal. The vagina may have a white discharge, which can persist for up to a week or more. On occasion, it may be tinged with blood (as a result of withdrawal of maternal hormones) during the first several days after delivery. An imperforate hymen may result in hydrometrocolpos, which may present as a lower abdominal or bulging mass that protrudes through the labia and requires decompression. Often, a hymenal tag is visible just at the vaginal orifice.

Males: In term boys, the penis is ~ 3–4 cm in length, and the scrotum will have rugae and pigmentation. Penile length < 2.5 cm is abnormal—proceed to endocrine workup! The prepuce is normally tight, adherent, and should not be forcibly retracted. Hypospadias is fairly common and may be present in a range—from a small ventral cleft at the distal end of the shaft to a major ventral defect along the length of the penis. Any degree of hypospadias is a contraindication to elective circumcision. Chordee, a "ventral bend" in the penis, commonly accompanies hypospadias. Epispadias can also occur on the dorsum of the penis, but this is much less common than hypospadias. Testes are usually in the scrotum but may be palpated in the upper scrotum, or even the inguinal canal. An undescended testicle will result in findings of less

notes

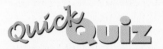

1) What is *diastasis recti*?

2) Describe an omphalocele.

3) How does gastroschisis differ from an omphalocele?

4) What is prune belly?

5) What does delayed separation of the umbilical cord possibly indicate?

6) True or False: Vaginal discharge is uncommon in the female neonate.

7) What is the lower limit of normal for penis size?

8) Impaction of meconium with resulting intestinal obstruction is common in what disease?

9) How do you screen for congenital dislocation of the hip?

rugae and other mature features of the affected side. Hydroceles are common in the scrotum and disappear gradually. A hydrocele that changes in size or persists is indicative of an indirect inguinal hernia, and peritoneal communication exists. Testicular torsion can occur in infancy and would manifest as an enlarged testicle with overlaying discoloration of the scrotum.

Ambiguous genitalia obviously require further investigation. The difficulty occurs in differentiating between a very enlarged clitoris and pigmented, fused labia vs. a very small penis with extensive hypospadias and a bifid scrotum. This is generally cause for an emergent genetic consult.

ANUS

Imperforate anus is one of the most common and important abnormalities to identify. It is not always obvious! It can occur with a simultaneous fistula that opens ventral to the normal anus, which may look like a "normal-appearing" anal dimple with no opening. Beware: Meconium presence does not rule out imperforate anus, since it could come via a fistula.

Meconium usually passes within the first 12 hours of birth, and 99% of term infants will pass meconium within the first 48 hours. Note: Impaction of meconium that causes intestinal obstruction (meconium ileus) is often associated with cystic fibrosis (CF)! Meconium ileus is also associated with small bowel atresia.

SPINAL COLUMN

Midline abnormalities include small dimples, tufts of hair, and pilonidal sinuses. These are discussed in further detail in the Neurology section. If noted, investigate carefully for seeping fluid. Midline cutaneous abnormalities can also indicate occult spina bifida or an entity known as diastematomyelia—the division of the spinal cord into 2 parts! This would eventually result in what is known as a "tethered cord." Note: Neural crest defects can occur and include meningoceles, myelomeningoceles, and rachischisis. These defects are more common among infants born in the late fall and early winter (suggesting an environmental influence) and are far less frequent when women of childbearing age receive folic acid supplementation. If there is a tumor of the spine at birth, it is almost always a teratoma.

EXTREMITIES

In the newborn, trauma and positional deformities are common. Fractures of the femur, humerus, and clavicles are the types of fractures you usually see. For most positional deformities, gentle pressure should restore the limb/joint to its normal configuration; corrective positioning or exercise/stretching should suffice. If it does not correct with gentle pressure, call for orthopedic evaluation.

Hips: If the hips are flexed to 90°, the legs normally can be abducted until the knees touch the table. If this cannot be done, or can be accomplished only unilaterally, you must consider congenital dislocation of the hip! With this condition, the head of the femur is displaced posteriorly and is out of the acetabular fossa. All daughters of affected mothers with developmental dysplasia of the hip should be screened aggressively. Note: Hip clicks can be felt in up to 10% of newborns, but only 10% of these are due to congenital hip dislocation! 2 ways to check for this:

1) Ortolani: Place the infant in the supine position. Place your thumb along the inner thigh while placing your index and middle fingers along the greater trochanter. With the hip flexed 90° and without rotation, gently abduct the hip while lifting the leg anteriorly. With a positive Ortolani, you feel a "clunk" as the femoral head reduces.

2) Barlow: Place the infant in supine position. Flex the hip 90°. Apply adduction and posteriorly directed pressure to the knee. With a positive test, you feel a "clunk" as the femoral head exits the acetabulum posteriorly. Infants in a breech position *in utero* tend to keep their hips flexed after birth. These infants, particularly girls, are at increased risk for hips that dislocate easily.

Limbs: Hemihypertrophy and hemiatrophy occur when the limbs are of different size but proportioned. Hemihypertrophy is sometimes associated with Wilms tumor, hepatoblastoma, and adrenal carcinoma. With phocomelia, there is an abnormal shape to the limb, which was common in infants of mothers who took thalidomide during pregnancy. Short limbs also will occur with achondroplastic and thanatophoric dysplasia. There is a condition called arthrogryposis multiplex congenita, in which the newborn has severe contractures of multiple joints. Amazingly, you can resolve these by simple, manual pressure.

notes

Syndactyly (fusion of digits) and polydactyly (extra digits) are fairly common. It is important to identify findings in the extremities, such as "clenched hand" with overriding index finger and rocker-bottom feet, both of which are seen in trisomy 18. Think "syndromes" when confronted with preaxial-duplications (thumb or great toe) in contrast to postaxial (pinkies) duplications.

Amniotic bands may wrap tightly around a limb and result in sharp, deep creases or depressions. They can also cause amputations of digits and obstruct lymphatic flow. Alternatively, amniotic bands can be swallowed, and the infant presents with atypical cleft lip.

NEUROLOGICAL EXAM

Mental Alertness

Alertness is marked by transient eye openings and movement of the face and extremities. The term newborn will frequently respond to auditory and visual stimuli. Irritability is noted when the infant cries spontaneously and cannot be consoled. Lethargy can be inferred if the infant does not respond to appropriate stimulation. Table 8-8 lists Prechtl states of sleep and wakefulness in the newborn. Note: State 3 is known as "quiet alertness"—the state when it is best to elicit good neurological responses.

Examination of cranial nerves and motor function follows pediatrics textbook standards.

6 important maneuvers, however, must be reviewed now:

1) Popliteal angle: The angle formed, at the knee, by doing the following: Flex the baby's thighs out and laterally beside the abdomen. Then extend the knee to its limit.

2) Foot dorsiflexion angle: Formed by extending the baby's knee, then dorsiflexing the ankle by moving the sole of the foot with your finger. Measure the angle between the dorsum of the foot and the anterior aspect of the leg.

3) Scarf sign: Pull the baby's hand across its chest toward the opposite shoulder, and note the position of the elbow.

4) Forearm recoil: Extend the baby's arm passively at the elbow by pulling the hand. Then, immediately release the hand and observe the speed of recoil.

5) Ventral flexion in the axis: Place the baby supine, grab the lower limbs, and push both legs and pelvis toward the head to look for maximum curvature of the spine.

6) Dorsal flexion in the axis: Lay the baby on his/her side. Pull both legs backward with one hand while resting your other hand on the baby's lumbar region. Normally, extension is minimal or absent.

Remember: For all of these, flexion always exceeds extension; it is considered abnormal if it does not.

Important on the Peds Board exam are the following "primitive" reflexes—ones that are almost always present in the newborn and don't wane until several months of age:

Moro Reflex: Hold the baby up off the bed by its hands in abduction, lift its shoulders a few inches off the bed, and then release the baby's hands. The normal response is for the baby to slap you. No! Wait! I mean, the normal response is for the baby to rapidly abduct and extend its arms, followed by complete opening of the hands.

Finger Grasp: Insert your fingers into the baby's hands to get flexion of its fingers around your fingers, then lift the baby while he/she holds on to your fingers with his/her palmar grasp.

Automatic Walking (sometimes called "stepping reflex"): Hold the baby upright with its feet on the table/bed in a standing position. Next, tilt the baby slightly forward. The baby should make a step forward.

Suck-swallow Reflex: Place your finger (clean, please) in the baby's mouth and note the strength and rhythm of sucking and its synchrony with swallowing. Notwithstanding the validity of this reflex assessment, I have to poke fun at the neurologist who came up with this. This person claims that you can estimate the number of movements in a burst, the rate, the negative pressure perceived, and the inter-burst time. For example, this same neurologist says that by 36 weeks gestation, a baby should have 8 or more movements in a burst, with 2 movements/second, "high" negative pressure, and an inter-burst time of 5–10 seconds! Yeah, sure.

What about standard tendon reflexes? The term infant will have normal biceps, knee, and ankle reflexes. It is also normal for an infant to have some clonus at the ankle. The Babinski sign is extensor (upgoing). Investigate any asymmetry or absence of reflexes.

Table 8-8: Prechtl States of Sleep and Wakefulness in the Newborn	
State	Findings
1	Eyes closed, regular respiration, no movements
2	Eyes closed, irregular respiration, no gross movements
3	Eyes open, no gross movements
4	Eyes open, gross movements, no crying
5	Crying, eyes can be open or closed

NEONATAL PROPHYLAXIS

EYE PROPHYLAXIS

Neonatal ophthalmia still occurs in the U.S. Usually, it is due to *Neisseria gonorrhoeae* and is prevented by instilling 2 drops of 1% silver nitrate, or by using a 1–2 cm ribbon of ointment that contains either 1% tetracycline or 0.5% erythromycin. Place either modality in each eye within 1 hour of birth. Rinsing the eyes afterwards is contraindicated, because it will reduce effectiveness of the treatment. Silver nitrate can cause a mild chemical conjunctivitis within 24–48 hours of instillation.

notes

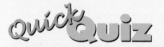

1) For most neurologic maneuvers, which should be more prominent: flexion or extension?

2) Describe the Moro reflex.

3) Describe the grasp reflex.

4) What standard tendon reflexes does a newborn have?

5) Is ankle clonus abnormal in a newborn?

6) What should an infant born to a hepatitis B surface antigen positive mother receive soon after delivery?

7) How is hypoglycemia evaluated in a newborn? What is the current "cut-off" value?

8) What screening test may a blood transfusion interfere with?

VITAMIN K

Give Vitamin K_1 as a 1 mg IM injection during the first few hours of birth to prevent hemorrhagic disease of the newborn. Oral dosing can be used but is discouraged because of its relative transient effect.

HEPATITIS B

Hepatitis B immunization is discussed in the Growth and Development/Preventive Pediatrics section. Remember: Give hepatitis B immune globulin, in addition to the vaccine, to infants born to mothers who are positive for hepatitis B surface antigen. The baby also should be cleaned thoroughly with a disinfectant before receiving any injection. If the mother is hepatitis B surface antigen positive, give the baby a 2nd dose of vaccine at 1 month of age, then the 3rd dose at 6 months of age.

CORD CARE

No single method of umbilical cord care has been proven to be superior in preventing colonization and disease. Common methods include the local application of antimicrobial agents, such as triple-dye, iodophor ointment, or hexachlorophene powder. Alcohol use alone is not effective in preventing umbilical cord colonization and omphalitis. Upon discharge home, the best care is to leave the umbilical stump exposed to air, swab it daily with a drying agent like alcohol, and avoid any moist coverings. Topical antibiotics are not routinely indicated.

CIRCUMCISION

Recent policy statements of the AAP stipulate that the medical benefits of circumcision do not warrant its routine use.

NEONATAL SCREENING

GLUCOSE

Routine glucose screening is no longer recommended. Screening should be directed toward those infants at risk for pathologic hypoglycemia:
• Born to mothers with diabetes
• Large for gestational age (LGA)
• Small for gestational age (SGA)
• Premature (< 37 weeks gestation)
• Low birth weight (< 2,500 g)
• Polycythemia (HCT > 70%)
• Hypothermia
• Low Apgar scores (< 5 at 1 minute)
• Stress (sepsis, respiratory distress, other abnormalities)

Also screen if any of these clinical signs are noted:
• Tremors, irritability
• High-pitched cry
• Lethargy, hypotonia
• Cyanosis, apnea, tachypnea
• Poor suck
• Jitteriness
• Seizures

If a screen shows a blood glucose < 40 mg/dL, send a serum/plasma glucose to the lab immediately, and treat the infant for hypoglycemia pending the confirmatory test result. 40 mg/dL is the new cut-off, as compared to the old 30 mg/dL.

HEMATOCRIT

Routine testing is no longer recommended, but it is frequently performed in many newborn nurseries.

BLOOD TYPE

If the mom's blood type is O or Rh negative, determine the infant's blood type, and do a direct Coombs test. Perform these same steps if the mother has a positive antibody titer.

INBORN ERRORS OF METABOLISM / HEMOGLOBINOPATHIES

Generally, all newborns in the U.S. are screened for hypothyroidism and phenylketonuria, and most states screen for galactosemia and sickle-cell disease. Depending on the state, the newborn may also be screened for cystic fibrosis, congenital adrenal hyperplasia, maple syrup urine disease, syphilis, and HIV. Other screenings may include infections, hemoglobinopathies, and metabolic diseases, depending on local laws. Errors can occur if the tests are done too quickly after birth (hypothyroidism) or following transfusion (hemoglobinopathies).

HEARING

Screening

The AAP recommends screening neonates. Two methods are available: the auditory brainstem response (ABR) and the otoacoustic emissions (OAE).

TOXIC SUBSTANCES / ILLICIT DRUGS

Most nurseries have specific guidelines for testing infants for these substances or drugs, based on maternal/paternal risk factors noted in the obstetrical history or symptoms the infant exhibits.

MULTIPLE BIRTHS

EPIDEMIOLOGY

The incidence of multiple births is increasing in the U.S. More than 2% of all births are now multiples (twins: 1/43; triplets: 1/13,000+); the majority are preterm and/or low-birth-weight infants. Note: Much of the increase in the "twinning rate" has occurred in mothers ages 40–49; these are mostly dizygous twins. Monozygous twinning has not increased in number.

PRENATAL ASSESSMENT

Prenatal assessment involves multiple factors, but the most important to the physician treating the infants is how extensive prenatal care has been for the mother. 20–50% of multiple gestations have preterm labor. Also, there is a slight increase in premature rupture of the membranes, pregnancy-induced hypertension, placenta previa, and polyhydramnios—compared to single births. Perform ultrasound at 18–20 weeks for multiple fetuses, and repeat every 3–4 weeks.

DELIVERY AND PERINATAL PROBLEMS

The most common delivery room complications with multiple births include malpresentation, umbilical cord compression, placental abruption, congenital abnormalities, and premature delivery. Triplets have an 85% chance of premature birth, with a mean birth weight of 1,700 grams. Around 80% of twin pregnancies result in vertex position of Twin A. Note: 50% of twins and 70% of triplets are delivered by C-section. With twins, fetal lung maturation is tested by sampling the amnionic fluid of the "least stressed" twin, which will usually be the non-presenting twin.

Risk for respiratory distress and necrotizing enterocolitis are the same for singletons and twins, as long as gestational age is the controlling factor.

Twins at greatest risk for delivery room complications are monoamniotic twins!

Congenital malformations are much more common in twins than in singletons. Nearly all twins have some abnormality related to positional crowding. Monozygous twins have a 6–10% risk of congenital malformation.

Conjoined twins occur in 1/50,000 births. This can occur only in monoamniotic, monochorionic twins. It occurs during the 3rd week of gestation, resulting from failure to separate. The most common fusion sites are the chest and abdomen.

Twin-to-twin transfusion: This occurs only in twins with a monochorionic placenta. Transfer of blood between twins occurs through AV connections in the placenta.

Fetal growth restriction: The growth rate for twins differs from that for singletons at 30 weeks gestation and is much more linear than the accelerated growth seen in singletons. Average gestational age for twins is 37 weeks, with a weight ≥ 2,400 grams. (As stated above, triplets have an 85% chance of premature delivery, with a mean weight of 1,700 grams.) Discordance of growth is defined as a difference of 20% between the weights of the twins. This is not a factor if the smaller twin weighs > 2,500 grams at birth. Intrauterine growth restriction (IUGR) is much more likely in triplets than in twins. Weight discordance in triplets occurs in > 2/3 of deliveries.

SMALL FOR GESTATIONAL AGE (SGA)

Infants who are small for gestational age (SGA) have birth weights < the 10th percentile for their gestational age. Intrauterine growth restriction (IUGR) is defined as a rate of growth less than the 5th percentile expected for a normal infant. Any insult/abnormality to the placenta or fetus can lead to growth reduction/failure. Low-birth-weight infants are defined as < 2,500 grams at birth; very low-birth-weight (VLBW) infants are defined as < 1,500 grams at birth; and extremely low-birth-weight (ELBW) infants are defined as < 1,000 grams at birth.

Whether an abnormality is intrinsic or extrinsic can be determined by whether the growth is symmetrically or asymmetrically abated. Intrinsic abnormalities frequently cause symmetrical growth problems, while extrinsic effects cause asymmetrical problems. These are discussed individually in other sections.

The SGA infant frequently presents with clinical problems at birth or soon after; these include:
- Asphyxia
- Temperature instability
- Glucose abnormalities (both hypo- and hyper-)
- Immune dysfunction
- Metabolism abnormalities (both protein and lipid)
- Neuro-developmental abnormalities
- Polycythemia-hyperviscosity

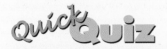

DIABETES IN PREGNANCY

Maternal hyperglycemia causes fetal hyperglycemia. This results in fetal pancreatic B-cell stimulation, with subsequent hyperinsulinemia.

Well-known complications include:
- Sudden fetal death in the 3rd trimester
- Macrosomia
- Birth trauma due to macrosomia/shoulder dystocia
- Increased rate of C-sections
- IUGR
- Hypoglycemia
- Hypocalcemia
- Hypomagnesemia
- Polycythemia
- Cardiomyopathy
- Congenital heart disease: septal defects, transposition of the great arteries, truncus arteriosus, coarctation
- Congenital abnormalities: lumbosacral dysgenesis/caudal regression
- Unconjugated hyperbilirubinemia
- Small left colon syndrome
- Renal anomalies

Additionally, we know that these infants have an increased risk of obesity and diabetes later in life.

Note: Infants of mothers with gestational diabetes only (onset only in pregnancy) are at increased risk for all of the above morbidities, except for congenital abnormalities and future obesity/diabetes.

Macrosomia increases the risk of birth trauma and C-section delivery. Infants of diabetic women have almost 2x as much fat, and an increase in nonfatty tissue, especially in the shoulder and intrascapular regions. The liver, heart, and other organs are enlarged. Brain size, however, is not increased. Excess fat appears to accumulate at > 30 weeks gestation. Even with effective insulin therapy for mothers with diabetes during pregnancy, 20–30% of their infants will still develop macrosomia.

Hypoglycemia in a neonate is defined as blood glucose < 40 mg/dL. It occurs during the first 24 hours in 25–50% of infants born to diabetic mothers. This is due to decreased production of glucose, as well as its increased clearance. The infant may present with lethargy, hypotonia, tremors, frank seizures, sweating, or cyanosis.

Hypocalcemia occurs in 10–20% of infants born to diabetic mothers. It is frequently not an isolated finding and occurs with hypophosphatemia, as well as hypomagnesemia. The mechanism is unclear, but some speculate it is due to the fact that parathormone concentrations are much lower in these newborns than in those of nondiabetic mothers. Abnormal placental function may also be a culprit. The hypomagnesemia is due to the increased renal losses seen in diabetics. Hypocalcemia may present as increased tremors, twitches, and frank convulsions. Note: Cardiac abnormalities can occur—particularly QT interval prolongation—but not as consistently as in older children. If asphyxia occurs at birth, give calcium gluconate with parenteral fluids during the first few days of life, because asphyxia increases the risk of hypocalcemia. If the infant is symptomatic with hypocalcemia, infuse him/her with 10% calcium gluconate at 2 mL/kg over 5 minutes. Cardiac monitoring is necessary during this infusion. If the infant is also hypomagnesemic, also give a 50% solution of magnesium at a dose of 0.25 mg/kg IM.

Hyperbilirubinemia occurs in ~ 30% of infants born to diabetics. This is likely due to the baby's large size and increased risk of birth trauma. The increased incidence of polycythemia also increases the prevalence of jaundice.

Polycythemia occurs in ~ 20% of infants born to diabetic mothers. This likely is responsible for the increased incidence of hyperviscosity in these infants.

Cardiomyopathy also occurs with increased frequency, presenting as thickening of the interventricular septum and one or both ventricular walls. This is likely due to the infant's intrauterine exposure to increased levels of insulin. Most of these infants are asymptomatic, with the finding showing up only on ECG or echocardiogram. Usually, the hypertrophy resolves by 3–6 months of age, and the infants are normal thereafter. Rarely, the septal thickening will be so marked as to cause left ventricular flow obstruction, resulting in CHF.

Hyaline membrane disease (also see later) occurs in ~ 10% of infants born to diabetic mothers. Insulin appears to block the development of enzymes necessary for the synthesis of lectin, which is a precursor of surfactant. Moreover, deposition of glycogen in lung interstitium may further compromise pulmonary function.

Congenital anomalies occur 2–4x more frequently in infants of diabetic mothers. The most common ones are ventricular septal defects, neural tube defects, gastrointestinal atresia, and urinary tract malformations. Note: If an infant presents with spinal agenesis associated with caudal regression syndrome, suspect that the infant's mother was diabetic! Another anomaly found usually only in infants of diabetic mothers is microcolon—neonatal, small left colon syndrome. It looks like gastrointestinal obstruction due to aganglionic megacolon, or even Hirschsprung disease. The clue will be that these infants have normal innervation of the bowel, and will eventually develop normal intestinal function.

What causes the increased risk of congenital anomalies in infants of diabetic mothers? Most likely, it is due to poor diabetes control before conception and during early pregnancy, when fetal organogenesis is occurring. Therefore, it is highly recommended that the mother's diabetes be controlled before pregnancy and to continue tight control during the first trimester.

What happens to these babies? Most infants born to diabetic mothers have an increased incidence of obesity later in life. They also have an increased incidence of diabetes by the time they are adolescents, because they appear to have impaired insulin responsiveness by this age. Much is still not understood, but many feel that a unique gender-correlated risk may exist—infants of fathers with insulin-dependent diabetes are at much higher risk of developing diabetes than infants of mothers with insulin-dependent diabetes.

RESPIRATORY DISEASES OF THE NEWBORN

RESPIRATORY DISTRESS SYNDROME HYALINE MEMBRANE DISEASE

Hyaline membrane disease (HMD) is the most common cause of respiratory failure in the newborn, occurring in 1–2% of all newborns. With improved therapy today, 85–95% of infants survive. The incidence of HMD is inversely related to gestational age. This means that 60–80% (but not 100%) of infants born < 28 weeks will develop HMD, while it rarely occurs in a term infant. Preterm, Caucasian males have the highest incidence. HMD is due to lack of surfactant and the lack of development of the alveoli, usually due to prematurity. The alveoli do not open properly, resulting in atelectasis, decreased functional residual capacity, and an inability to ventilate the lungs, and thus, leading to hypoxemia and tissue hypoxia.

The major constituents of surfactant are dipalmitoylphosphatidylcholine (lecithin), phosphatidylglycerol, apoproteins (surfactant proteins SP-A, B, C, D), and cholesterol. Lecithin makes up 65% of surfactant. As gestational age increases, more surfactant is synthesized and stored in Type II alveolar cells [Know]. Mature levels of pulmonary surfactant occur at > 35 weeks.

Besides premature birth, other factors increase the risk of developing HMD:
• Male sex
• Hypothermia
• Fetal distress/asphyxia
• Caucasian race
• C-section
• Diabetic mother
• Second-born twin
• Family history of HMD

Other factors actually reduce the risk:
• Maternal hypertension
• Premature rupture of membranes
• Sub-acute placental abruption
• Maternal use of narcotics

Predicting which infant may develop HMD can be done with the use of the lecithin-sphingomyelin (L/S) ratio in amnionic fluid. Concentrations of lecithin and sphingomyelin are nearly equal during the mid-second trimester, but by 34 weeks, lecithin is twice as prominent as sphingomyelin—indicating maturation of lung tissue. This ratio is used to determine adequate lung maturity. Also, we know that prenatal administration of betamethasone or dexamethasone will result in decreased incidence and severity of HMD. Therefore, give either of these agents at 24–34 weeks gestation to women at significant risk for preterm birth (generally, ruptured membranes or significant inappropriate cervical effacement). 2 doses of 12 mg of betamethasone IM 24 hours apart, or 4 doses of 6 mg dexamethasone given IM 12 hours apart, is recommended. Administer the first dose of intratracheal surfactant as soon as possible at delivery.

Clinically, HMD can present as early as the first few minutes of life, but may not be recognized until several hours after birth. Usually, the key feature will be tachypnea > 60 breaths per minute. Grunting, nasal flaring, intracostal/subcostal retractions, decreased capillary refill, and poor skin color will also frequently be noted. If it progresses, respiratory failure may occur, requiring aggressive interventions. The signs and symptoms will usually peak at ~ 3 days and then improve gradually or rapidly, depending on the severity of the underlying damage. Recovery is frequently heralded by diuresis. In infants weighing < 1,500 grams, a shunt may develop through a patent ductus arteriosus if pulmonary vascular resistance falls rapidly as systemic arterial resistance rises. This will result in pulmonary edema and require treatment with prostaglandin inhibitors or ligation. Mortality most frequently occurs on days 2–7, due to alveolar air leaks and pulmonary or intraventricular hemorrhage.

Diagnosis: Generally, this is a clinical diagnosis with supporting evidence from radiologic and blood gas values. The CXR will be normal early but, by 6–12 hours, an air bronchogram will show a fine, reticular granularity (often described as "ground glass" haziness). The blood gases will show hypoxemia early on, with the development of hypercarbia

notes

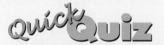
and metabolic acidosis. Group B streptococcus is probably the most commonly entertained diagnosis in the differential. Congenital heart disease also must be considered, as well as numerous lung abnormalities.

Treatment: Since most of these infants have low birth weights, follow general guidelines. Maintain core temperatures at 36.5–37° C (97.7–98.6° F). Provide IV fluids/nutrition. Give 10% glucose in the first 24 hours at a rate of 60–75 mL/kg/24 hours. Dopamine may be needed to support blood pressure if fluids alone are not adequate. After 24 hours, add electrolytes and increase fluid volumes to 120–150 mL/kg/24 hour. Provide oxygen to keep arterial oxygen levels of 55–70 mmHg. If oxygen measured by PaO_2 cannot be kept > 50, attempt CPAP at a pressure of 6–10 cm H_2O by nasal prongs. If CPAP is ineffective in keeping oxygen levels > 50, intubate with mechanical ventilation. Rates of 60–80 breaths/min, with a short inspiratory time of only 0.2–0.3 seconds with synchronization, appear to minimize pulmonary air leak. Control of $PaCO_2$ appears to be less important, and many will let the $PaCO_2$ remain > 50 mmHg. High-frequency oscillatory ventilation in these infants is controversial, and 2 trials have shown increased risk of intraventricular hemorrhage with such intervention. Additional potential complications include pneumothorax, patent ductus and, following recovery, bronchopulmonary dysplasia.

Prophylax infants < 28 weeks gestation with surfactant therapy in the delivery room. Older infants may be similarly treated if they meet criteria established by the organizations and hospitals involved. Most consider an infant who requires > 50% FiO_2 to maintain a PaO_2 > 50 mmHg as a candidate for surfactant therapy.

TRANSIENT TACHYPNEA OF THE NEWBORN

Transient tachypnea of the newborn has gone through several permutations of names, including syndrome of retained fetal lung liquid, persistent postnatal pulmonary edema, and respiratory distress syndrome Type II. It usually occurs in a term infant after a precipitous vaginal or, more typically, a C-section delivery. Most infants present with tachypnea and may have grunting, with some developing cyanosis requiring brief oxygen administration.

The lung examination is usually clear, with CXR showing prominent pulmonary vasculature, fluid in the fissures, flattening of the diaphragms due to overaeration, and occasional pleural fluid. In contrast to HMD, air bronchograms and reticular granularity are absent on CXR.

The signs/symptoms usually resolve by day 3–4 of life. Most lung liquid is resorbed within 24 hours of birth. Oxygen may be required, but usually no further interventions or therapies are necessary. Diuretics are not indicated.

PERSISTENT PULMONARY HYPERTENSION OF THE NEWBORN (PPHN)

Persistent pulmonary hypertension of the newborn (PPHN) is not a specific disease but a syndrome due to various etiologies.

The most commonly identified etiologies:
• Meconium aspiration
• Pulmonary infections
• HMD
• Sepsis
• Pulmonary hypoplasia
• Hyperviscosity/polycythemia
• Hypoglycemia
• Hypothermia

Many etiologies are idiopathic! Affected infants have no evidence of parenchymal lung disease. It occurs in from 1/500 to 1/1,500 births, most commonly in term infants without congenital anomalies.

Remember: A dramatic change occurs in the pulmonary circulation after birth. In utero, the pulmonary circulation is a high-resistance circuit; immediately after delivery, this drops to a low-resistance circuit. This drop must occur so that the pulmonary blood flow can increase 8–10-fold to allow adequate gas exchange in the lung. If this does not occur, the infant has postnatal persistence of right-to-left ductal shunting (through a patent ductus arteriosus) or right-to-left atrial shunting (through patent foramen ovale). Both result in severe hypoxemia, which will be refractory to oxygen administration (clue for the Boards!) or very labile oxygen requirements, because pulmonary vascular resistance oscillates.

notes

Clinically, symptoms usually appear in the first 12 hours of life, frequently in the delivery room. Tachypnea with cyanosis is the most common feature. A key is that hypoxia is frequently much more severe than the findings indicated on the CXR! Hypoxia, hypercapnia, and acidosis often act to worsen pulmonary artery vasoconstriction. Another clue: Differential cyanosis. Greater oxygen saturation in the upper body compared to the lower body is classic for PPHN, due to right-to-left ductus arteriosus shunting. You will hear a tricuspid regurgitation murmur (precordial systolic murmur), as well as a loud, second heart sound (P2).

Echocardiogram is the easiest path to diagnosis. You see elevated pulmonary artery pressure and the atrial septum being pulled to the left, with right-to-left shunting of blood across the ductus arteriosus or the foramen ovale. A cardiac catheterization can confirm the diagnosis. Other differentials to consider on the Board exam: Total anomalous pulmonary venous return (plus other congenital cyanotic heart disease) and the etiologies that predispose to PPHN, like hypoglycemia, sepsis, and polycythemia.

Direct treatment at the underlying etiology, if one exists, and correct tissue hypoxia. Mechanical ventilation is frequently required, and, in the past, tolazoline was used to non-selectively vasodilate (as an alpha-adrenergic antagonist) the pulmonary arterial system. We don't use tolazoline much anymore because of the effect on systemic pressures. Hyperventilation is also used, lowering the PCO_2 which, in turn, causes decreased pulmonary vasoconstriction. You also can try pressors (dopamine/dobutamine) to reverse the ductal shunt by elevating systemic blood pressure. Sedation is useful to avoid the infant struggling against the ventilator and further increasing intrathoracic and pulmonary pressures. Inhaled nitrous oxide reduces the need for extracorporeal membrane oxygenation (ECMO). Note: Methemoglobinemia is a complication of inhaled nitrous oxide! Use ECMO when mechanical ventilation, drug therapy, and 100% oxygen do not alleviate the PPHN. It is reportedly necessary in 5–10% of patients with PPHN.

MECONIUM ASPIRATION

Meconium aspiration is one of the most common etiologies of respiratory failure in newborns. The presence of meconium in the amniotic fluid should be considered as a sign of fetal distress. Meconium staining can be found in up to 5–15% of term and post-term births. Around 1/3 will require mechanical ventilation. The mortality rate for all infants with meconium aspiration is 4–5%.

The AAP and its neonatal resuscitation guidelines now recommend direct tracheal suction only in those infants whose breathing is depressed at birth and have meconium staining.

Clinically, the infant presents with signs of respiratory distress shortly after a meconium-complicated delivery, with tachypnea, intercostal retractions and, frequently, cyanosis. On physical examination, the neonate will have a barrel-shaped chest, a distended abdomen, and coarse, upper airway breath sounds. The CXR will frequently show patchy infiltrates; pneumothoraces are common (the result of a "ball-valve" effect caused by particulate meconium plugs that lead to air trapping).

During the first hour after birth, infants are frequently hypoxemic with metabolic acidosis. Supplemental oxygen is usually required, and mechanical ventilation is necessary as the infant's PCO_2 rises and air exchange becomes severely compromised. Pneumothoraces and pneumomediastinum are very common (~ 15%) in mechanically ventilated infants. PPHN also is a common complication (see above), as are bacterial infections and chemical pneumonia. The problem is that infection is difficult to confirm with everything else going on. Use of prophylactic antibiotics has not been shown to improve outcomes and likely increases risk of developing a resistant organism. Usually, the prognosis is complicated by the degree of asphyxia that has occurred and also by the resulting damage to the brain, heart, liver, and kidneys.

PNEUMOTHORAX AND PNEUMOMEDIASTINUM

Asymptomatic, unilateral pneumothorax is really quite common, occurring in around 1–2% of newborns. Symptomatic pneumothorax and pneumomediastinum are rarer, with pneumomediastinum (many asymptomatic) reported in ~ 0.25% of newborns. In some infants, mediastinal air dissects into the subcutaneous tissues around the neck, causing subcutaneous emphysema. Pneumothorax and pneumomediastinum occur more commonly in infants with underlying lung disease, as you would expect.

Clinical signs and symptoms depend a lot on how big the leak is and where it is located. Symptomatic infants will usually present with respiratory distress, which could be as simple as just an increased respiratory rate—or as serious as full-blown severe dyspnea. Tachycardia, hypotension, and cyanosis may also be present, depending on the degree of insult. Remember: Intrathoracic structures, like the heart, will be shifted toward the normal side and away from the pneumothorax. The diaphragm on the affected side is displaced downward; and if it is a right-sided pneumothorax, the liver also may be displaced downward.

Diagnose with a CXR; the leak is usually easy to see unless it is very small or the lung is stiff. It is usually easiest to see on an expiratory film (hey, little baby, take a deep breath and exhale fully. OK, this usually doesn't happen). With a tension pneumothorax, the heart and diaphragm deviation will usually be more prominent.

Since most pneumothoraces do not cause respiratory distress or significant problems, watchful waiting is usually the treatment. Most will resolve without intervention. If the pneumothorax is compromising the infant, immediately decompress with a 22-gauge Angiocath connected to a 3-way

notes

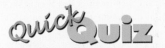

stopcock and a large syringe. Place the needle at the mid-clavicular line over the second intercostal space, and then advance it until it enters the pleural space. It is important to keep negative pressure on the syringe while advancing the needle. Once in the pleural space, remove the needle and leave in the catheter with the stopcock and syringe attached to the catheter in the pleural space. If the pneumothorax remains > 20% or the infant is still hypoxic or in distress, insert a chest tube. A pneumomediastinum usually does not require therapy unless the child is severely compromised.

PULMONARY HEMORRHAGE IN THE NEWBORN

Pulmonary hemorrhage is fairly common and occurs in approximately 1/1,000 live births. However, such hemorrhages are noted in 10–15% of autopsies of neonates. Most of these infants weigh < 2,500 grams. The mortality rate is very high in the neonatal period, and prematurity is the most common risk factor. Other risk factors include perinatal asphyxia and bleeding disorders. Clinically, it is a nightmare—the infant presents with blood oozing from the nose and mouth and is in severe respiratory distress. Immediate therapy includes tracheal suction, oxygen, and providing positive-pressure ventilation to maintain a high, positive expiratory pressure of at least 6–10 cm H_2O. It is important

to correct any underlying bleeding disorders or other correctable factors. Mortality is extremely high, but if the infant survives, there are usually no long-term pulmonary deficits.

INTERSTITIAL PULMONARY FIBROSIS (WILSON-MIKITY SYNDROME)

Interstitial pulmonary fibrosis is seen in infants without a history of hyaline membrane disease, who are < 32 weeks gestation, and with birth weight < 1,500 grams. It is rather gradual in onset over the first month of life. Dyspnea, tachypnea, and cyanosis develop slowly. Cough and wheezing may develop, but fever is usually not a factor. Lung collapse can occur, as well as right-sided heart failure. Symptoms increase over a 3–6 week period and persist for several months. They then gradually resolve—or the infant becomes progressively worse and develops respiratory and cardiac failure.

The CXR is classic: Early on, bilateral reticular infiltrates occur with development of multi-cystic lesions. The cysts enlarge and eventually come together to form a hyperlucent, bubble-like appearance. The CXR then gradually shows clearing over months and years. Treatment includes supplemental oxygen, bronchodilators, diuretics, and mechanical ventilation, if needed.

GROUP B STREPTOCOCCUS PNEUMONIA

Unlike some other bacterial pathogens, group B streptococcus pneumonia is exclusively a disease of the newborn age group. Infections with *Streptococcus agalactiae* (group B streptococcus = GBS) are usually grouped by age of onset and present quite differently. Early onset is defined as < 7 days of life; late onset is usually defined as 3–4 weeks of age. Early onset by far is the most common type of infection, and has been reported to occur in 2–4 cases/1,000 births. This rate increases 10x in mothers with known colonization. The early-onset form of the disease presents with pneumonia, sepsis, and occasionally meningitis. The late-onset form presents with sepsis and meningitis, and sometimes, focal infections (bone, etc.).

GBS colonize the birth canal and are transmitted to infants either by ascending infection *in utero* or during delivery. Ascending infection occurs more frequently if there has been prolonged rupture of membranes. Other risk factors for infection include premature birth, history of a prior infant with GBS infection, GBS in maternal urine (can just be colonization), and maternal fever.

In ~ 75% of early-onset GBS infections, there is a maternal risk factor (prolonged rupture of membranes, maternal fever, or chorioamnionitis). Most infants present early in life, at 8–12 hours of age. Respiratory symptoms predominate, with tachypnea and retractions most common. Cyanosis, apnea, poor perfusion, hypotension, and signs of sepsis follow

notes

quickly. When death occurs, it is due to progressive tissue hypoxia and shock. Laboratory values frequently show a severe leukopenia and thrombocytopenia, along with an abnormal PT/PTT. Usually, the organism can be readily cultured from the blood and tracheal secretions. Latex agglutination tests also can be used for rapid identification. Note: On the Board exam, if you're given a "normal, healthy" infant who has a +GBS antigen on a bagged urine, do not think he/she has invasive GBS! This is colonization and does not need further workup in an otherwise healthy infant.

Prevention: [Know] The gist of the latest (2002) guidelines is discussed on pg 8-4, and they are summarized in Table 8-9. This is a very testable area!

So, here are some practice scenarios/treatments:
1) Onset of labor is at 35 weeks gestation and GBS screening is negative: no prophylaxis.
2) Onset of labor is at 32 weeks gestation and GBS screening is positive; tocolysis is given to stop labor and it does so at 24 hours; labor resumes at 35 weeks and mother delivers a healthy boy: Start PCN IV for 48 hours, during and after tocolysis, at 32 weeks; stop PCN at the end of 48 hours, then resume it when mother goes into labor at 35 weeks; continue until delivery occurs.

Now, assume mom has been given appropriate prophylaxis. What do you do for the infant when he/she is born?
• If the baby has signs of sepsis, do the obvious workup and start therapy.
• If the mother received prophylaxis and the infant is < 35 weeks gestation, do a limited evaluation—observe for at least 48 hours in the hospital and proceed to full sepsis workup, if indicated.
• If the mother received prophylaxis and the infant is > 35 weeks, you must find out if the prophylaxis was started longer than 4 hours ago. If it was not (i.e., begun < 4 hours ago), just observe the infant for 48 hours in the hospital and institute a septic workup if signs/symptoms indicate a problem.
• If gestation is > 35 weeks and the time since prophylaxis was started is > 4 hours, don't do anything different for the infant, as compared to an infant of a non-GBS-colonized mother. This infant could go home as soon as 24 hours if everything is OK.

Considering all of this, what has effective prophylaxis and therapy achieved? It has reduced early-onset GBS disease by > 70%!

Treatment of GBS pneumonia/sepsis: For infants < 1 week of age, give PCN G IV in doses of 250,000–450,000 units/kg divided q 8 hours for initial therapy—until you rule out meningitis. For infants > 1 week of age, give daily doses of 450,000 units/kg divided q 6 hours. You also may use ampicillin in infants < 7 days at 200 mg/kg divided q 8 hours. For those > 7 days of age, dose is 300 mg/kg divided q 4 to 6 hours. Duration of therapy for isolated bacteremia is 10 days. Pneumonia usually requires 10–14 days of therapy. For uncomplicated meningitis, therapy is 14–21 days. Some recommend repeating the lumbar puncture at the end of therapy.

PATENT DUCTUS ARTERIOSUS

Patent ductus arteriosus (PDA) is discussed further in the Cardiology section.

The incidence of PDA is inversely related to the maturity of the infant and is common in infants with HMD complicated by hypoxemia. The best way to diagnose this condition is by echocardiogram. Signs specific for a PDA are a continuous murmur in both systole and diastole or hyperactive left ventricular impulse, but these findings are not as common as Board tests make you think. However, if the Board exam presents an infant with a continuous murmur and worsening respiratory status during the newborn period, put PDA high on your list! Other clues to look for: systolic heart murmur ("continuous" again is the buzz-word), hyperdynamic precordium, bounding peripheral pulses, a wide pulse pressure, and worsening respiratory status. ECG and CXR may not help much although the CXR may show some degree of cardiomegaly and/or pulmonary edema.

Treatment is institution-dependent and patient-specific. Some advocate conservative measures, such as fluid restriction, diuretics, and digitalis, but these have been found to not be effective. Using positive, end-expiratory pressure has been useful in

Table 8-9: Group B Streptococcus Preventative Guidelines
Women who should receive prophylaxis
GBS positive from vaginal/rectal cultures at 35–37 weeks
History of +GBS urine ($\geq 10^3$ colonies) at any time during her pregnancy
Previous Hx of infant born with invasive GBS disease
If cultures are not available/known and one of the following:
< 37 weeks gestation
$\geq$ 18 hours for membrane rupture
Fever of $\geq$ 100.4° F (38.0° C)
Women who do not need prophylaxis
Negative vaginal/rectal GBS screen in late gestation, regardless of intrapartum risk factors
Previous pregnancy with +GBS screen but current pregnancy screen is negative
GBS+ women with planned C-section before rupture of membranes

notes

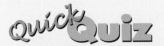

Quick Quiz

1) A healthy neonate is ready to be discharged. You note that a "bagged" urine has 10,000 colonies of *S. agalactiae* on culture. What should you do?

2) Know Table 8-9.

3) On the Board exam, you are presented an infant with a continuous murmur and worsening respiratory symptoms. What cardiac condition should you suspect?

4) What are the contraindications for indomethacin use?

5) Which infants may be predisposed to meconium plugs?

6) Meconium ileus with resulting obstruction should make you think of what autosomal recessive disorder?

7) What word describes the abdominal examination in a newborn with meconium ileus? What causes this?

8) What will the KUB show in an infant with meconium ileus-induced peritonitis?

9) How is meconium ileus usually treated?

managing infants with PDA. The amount of left-to-right shunt through the PDA decreases and systemic blood flow increases. Also, correct anemia. If the infant is symptomatic, you can do PDA ligation in the NICU; indomethacin is equally effective. The side effects of indomethacin therapy are oliguria and dilutional hyponatremia, which may require a halt to therapy. An additional serious complication is intestinal perforation.

When do you not use indomethacin?
When the infant has any of the following:
• Necrotizing enterocolitis
• Serum creatinine > 1.6 mg/dL ~~vs 1.8?~~
• Hourly urine output < 1 mL/kg
• Bleeding diathesis
• Platelets < 50,000 ~~vs 60,000~~

Interestingly, it is OK to use it if the infant has an interventricular hemorrhage! Indomethacin loses its effectiveness fairly quickly, and, by 3–4 days, it is less effective because prostaglandins play a less significant role in keeping the PDA open.

GASTROINTESTINAL DISORDERS IN NEWBORNS

MECONIUM PLUGS

Meconium plugs occur in the lower colon or anorectal region and are associated with lower-than-normal water content in the intestines. Meconium plugs can cause intestinal obstruction, ulceration, and perforation.

These types of plugs occur more commonly in infants with
• small left colon syndrome,
• cystic fibrosis,
• hypothyroidism,
• rectal aganglionosis,
• maternal drug abuse, and
• magnesium sulfate therapy for preeclampsia.

It may be prudent also to look for Hirschsprung disease. The plug usually can be relieved by using isotonic sodium solutions or diatrizoate sodium (Gastrografin®) enemas. These draw fluid rapidly into the intestinal lumen and allow the meconium plug to become loosened from the walls. It then can pass more easily.

Note: After the plug passes, observe the infant for presence of congenital aganglionic megacolon.

MECONIUM ILEUS

Meconium ileus is a lower intestinal obstruction that results from impactions due to meconium. Around 50% are simple intestinal obstruction; the others can be complicated by volvulus, intestinal atresia, or perforation. If you see this on the exam, be suspicious of cystic fibrosis! (What happens is that, in infants with CF, their meconium has an increased amount of albumin that makes it thick and viscid. This leads to obstruction at the level of the terminal ileum.)

The infant with meconium ileus will present with abdominal distention, vomiting of bilious material, and failure to pass a meconium stool. Classically, the abdomen is described as "doughy," because the bowel loops are filled with meconium instead of air.

A plain film of the abdomen usually will show distention of the proximal bowel, and occasionally, the right lower abdomen will have a "soap bubble" appearance. This is due to air mixing with the meconium. Meconium peritonitis can develop and may even be silent. It can be seen on CT scan as intraabdominal calcifications. A simple KUB will show the calcifications of meconium peritonitis (may also be seen *in utero*).

Simple meconium ileus can usually be treated without surgical intervention. Diatrizoate sodium enemas are used under fluoroscopy and refluxed into the terminal ileum. This will draw fluid into the bowel and allow the sticky mess to pass. Be careful, though. You have to watch the infant's electrolytes closely, because diatrizoate sodium is hyperosmolar and could push the infant into shock if there is too much fluid loss/redistribution. If the infant has meconium ileus that is complicated by intestinal atresia, volvulus, or perforation, you would usually order a laparotomy. Investigate cystic fibrosis by sweat test or genetic testing in all infants with meconium ileus or small bowel atresia.

notes

NECROTIZING ENTEROCOLITIS

Necrotizing enterocolitis (NEC) is an inflammatory lesion of the bowel characterized by abdominal distention, feeding difficulties, and GI bleeding, which can progress to intestinal gangrene with perforation and/or peritonitis. It is mainly a disease of preterm infants and is the most common intestinal emergency occurring in this age group. The distal ileum and proximal colon are most commonly affected. Asphyxia, polycythemia, hypertonic milk products, too-rapid feeding protocols, and various intestinal infections may predispose to mucosal injury and resulting bowel necrosis. Human milk has been shown to reduce the incidence of NEC. Cases will frequently occur in clusters in an NICU, suggesting an infectious etiology. Common organisms include *Clostridium perfringens*, *Escherichia coli*, *Staphylococcus epidermidis*, and rotavirus; but most cases have no identifiable infectious etiology.

NEC usually presents in the first 2 weeks of life; but in infants < 1,000 grams, it may occur up to 3 months of age. Abdominal distention will appear first. Bloody stools are seen in ~ 25% of cases. The spectrum of disease varies from mild, with just heme-positive stools, to full-blown sepsis/perforation and resulting death. A palpable abdominal mass and cellulitis may occur. Other clinical signs include emesis, increased gastric residual following feeds, and, as the disease progresses, abdominal wall erythema, bilious vomiting, lethargy, temperature instability, disseminated intravascular coagulation, and shock.

A classic finding on plain abdominal films is pneumatosis intestinalis—air in the wall of the bowel. If you see this on the films, it is pathognomonic. In the real world, it shows up ~ 50–75% of the time! An ominous sign is air in the hepatic portal system.

Diatrizoate sodium enema may show the pneumatosis intestinalis, and it is used if you cannot rule out congenital obstruction or midgut volvulus. Ultrasound may help you look for portal vein air if the plain film doesn't show it.

Treatment is rapid and involves nasogastric decompression, intravenous fluids, and stopping all enteral feeds to correct any metabolic/electrolyte derangements. Begin total parenteral nutrition and IV antibiotics after cultures are taken, usually ampicillin or an anti-pseudomonal PCN (ticarcillin, piperacillin) with gentamicin.

Remove umbilical catheters. Mechanical ventilation is frequently necessary. It is very important to isolate the infant from others in the NICU; if an epidemic is occurring, move affected infants away from non-affected infants.

A surgery consult is usually recommended early on, and exploratory laparotomy with resection of necrotic bowel and external ostomy is frequently required. Medical management works 75% of the time, but in the other 25%, the death rate is anywhere from 10% to 25%. Medical management usually requires 10–14 days, with parenteral feeding required throughout that time. Surgery is recommended for intestinal perforation with free air in the peritoneal space, cellulitis of the abdominal wall, or a peritoneal tap showing feces or pus. If the infant does not respond to medical management and has worsening acidosis or thrombocytopenia, exploratory laparotomy may be required to determine gangrenous bowel.

HYPERBILIRUBINEMIA (NEWBORN JAUNDICE)

Overview

Jaundice results from the deposition of excess bilirubin in the skin and sclerae, the latter of which usually are the most visible. "Physiologic" jaundice occurs because newborns have an increased rate of bilirubin production (mainly because of the shorter life span of their RBCs) and a decreased rate of bilirubin elimination (due to decreased ability of the newborn liver to conjugate bilirubin). Around 60% of newborns will become clinically jaundiced. Because more and more newborns are breastfed, the epidemiology of hyperbilirubinemia of the newborn has changed. Now, the peak bilirubin level is close to 4 days (instead of 3), and may not decline before day 6 or 7. For term bottle-fed newborns, the serum bilirubin level will peak at ~ 6 mg/dL. Normal levels (or the 95th percentile) for newborns peak at ~ 15–18 mg/dL.

The main source of bilirubin is the breakdown of hemoglobin from RBCs. Heme is degraded by heme oxygenase, which then results in the release of iron and the formation of CO and biliverdin. Biliverdin is then reduced to bilirubin by biliverdin reductase. At this point, bilirubin enters the liver and is changed to its excretable conjugated form. From the liver, it goes to the intestinal lumen. Here, it is either excreted or broken down by intestinal bacteria back into deconjugated bilirubin and resorbed into the blood stream.

The problem today is that most newborns are discharged from the hospital by 2 days of life. Therefore, a favorite question on the Boards would be to ask about a child who is home at day 4 of life and turning yellow. The infant to look for on the exam (and in real life) is a breastfed male, < 38 weeks gestation, and discharged at < 72 hours of age. Because of this change in practices, where babies are discharged before their peak bilirubin level will occur, many have switched to an "hour-specific," serum-bilirubin concentration instead of relying on "days of life." The "rate of rise" is an important factor to consider.

Specifically, which newborns should be checked? Order either a serum total bilirubin or a transcutaneous bilirubin on any newborn with clinical jaundice during the first 24 hours of life. Jaundice on the first day of life is always pathologic and requires evaluation for an associated infection. Also, any newborn you are sending home before the maximum serum bilirubin has been reached should probably be screened. You would then plot the value on a nomogram, according to the newborn's age in hours. This nomogram will help determine if the infant is at risk for being > 95th percentile down the road. Note: Intervention is urgent when the serum total bilirubin is > 25–30 mg/dL; do an exchange transfusion if it goes to > 30 mg/dL—or if the newborn has signs of kernicterus—see Table 8-10. (More on kernicterus below.)

notes

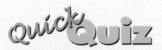

Quick Quiz

1) Which infants are more likely to have NEC?

2) What is the classic x-ray finding with NEC?

3) If you see air in the hepatic system in a patient with NEC, is this a good thing or a bad thing?

4) Describe the immediate management of an infant with suspected NEC.

5) When does the serum bilirubin peak occur in the healthy newborn?

6) Which newborns should you check or bring back for bilirubin checks?

7) Know the intervention and bilirubin levels to initiate therapy for hyperbilirubinemia.

8) Know Table 8-10.

9) What etiologies are common causes of hyperbilirubinemia from day of life 3–7? After the first week? For a more persistent time?

Breast-milk jaundice is common and is probably due to an increase in enterohepatic circulation—and may be because of an increased amount of β-glucuronidase (an inhibitor of bilirubin conjugation) in breast milk. It can remain for months.

What are the risk factors for severe hyperbilirubinemia?
- Pre-discharge total serum bilirubin in a high-risk zone defined as > 95th percentile for age
- Jaundice within the first 24 hours of life
- Hemolytic disease due to immune-mediated hemolysis
- Gestational age 35–36 weeks
- Previous sibling who required phototherapy
- Cephalohematoma
- Significant bruising from birth trauma

Table 8-10: Kernicterus
(adapted from Dennery, et al. NEJM 344;8:581-590, 2001)
2 FORMS: ACUTE AND CHRONIC
Acute
Phase 1 (occurs days 1–2): poor suckling, stupor, hypotonia, seizures
Phase 2 (middle of 1st week): hypertonia of extensor muscles, pisthotonus, retrocollis, fever
Phase 3 (after Phase 2): hypertonia
Chronic
First year of life: hypotonia, active deep-tendon reflexes, obligatory tonic neck reflexes, delayed motor skills

- An infant who is exclusively breastfed and has lost > 12% of body weight
- East Asian or Greek race

Other minor risk factors include:
- Gestational age 37–38 weeks
- Maternal age ≥ 25 years
- Male sex

"Protective factors" from developing hyperbilirubinemia include:
- Gestational age ≥ 41 weeks
- African-American race
- Exclusive bottle feeding

To make it simple, think of the pathologic causes of jaundice as due to 1 of 2 factors: increased bilirubin production or decreased elimination of bilirubin. The decreased elimination of bilirubin is a less common etiology than increased production. There are 3 main causes of decreased bilirubin destruction/elimination: impaired conjugation of bilirubin, deficiency in hepatic uptake, and increased enterohepatic circulation of bilirubin. Most of these have some sort of genetic basis. A common example is Gilbert syndrome—where there is decreased hepatic uptake of bilirubin and which displays varying expression in infants. Asian infants have an increased risk of having a DNA sequence variant that results in an amino acid change in the UDPGT (uridine diphosphate glucuronosyltransferase) protein. This also results in decreased uptake of bilirubin. Another rare (though not on the Boards!) syndrome to consider is Crigler-Najjar syndrome, Type I; this syndrome means an almost complete deficiency of UDPGT. Bilirubin encephalopathy occurs in the first days or months of life! Type II presents with less severe deficiency of UDPGT and, in contrast to Type I, responds to enzyme induction with phenobarbital; serum bilirubin values are rarely > 20 mg/dL.

Most of the common pathologic etiologies for hyperbilirubinemia in neonates are going to be problems with increased production of bilirubin. Consider causes of hemolysis as the etiology here:
- Blood-group incompatibilities; e.g., Rh, ABO, minor group antigens
- RBC enzyme deficiency; e.g., G6PD, pyruvate kinase
- Structural defects of the RBCs; e.g., spherocytosis

In premature infants, also note that RBC lifespan is shortened. Infants of diabetic mothers can exhibit hyperbilirubinemia due to either polycythemia or ineffective erythropoieses.

Determining when the jaundice started can be helpful. Jaundice that appears after the 3rd day during the first week suggests:
- Sepsis
- Urinary tract infections
- Congenital infection (syphilis, CMV)

If the jaundice occurs after the first week, consider:
- Breast-milk jaundice
- Sepsis
- Galactosemia
- Hypothyroidism
- CF
- Congenital atresia of the biliary ducts
- Hepatitis
- Spherocytosis
- Some other weird hemolytic anemia, like pyruvate kinase deficiency

Also, don't forget about drugs as an etiology, especially if the infant has something like G6PD deficiency.

If the jaundice is persistent, you have to think of the following:
- Inspissated bile syndrome
- Hyperalimentation/drug-induced cholestasis
- Hepatitis
- A TORCH disease
- Congenital atresia of the bile ducts
- Galactosemia

What do you do if the serum bilirubin is elevated in the jaundiced infant? You need to determine if it is a direct or indirect hyperbilirubinemia. If it is indirect, and there is reticulocytosis and a peripheral smear showing RBC destruction, consider hemolysis due to blood-group or other blood incompatibility as the likely etiology. If there is no blood-group incompatibility, suspect a nonimmunologic etiology, such as internal hemorrhage or polycythemia. For direct hyperbilirubinemia (bilirubin > 2 mg/dL) consider biliary atresia, choledochal cyst, cholestasis, hepatitis, inborn errors of metabolism, CF, and infections.

Treatment

For full-term infants with no evidence of hemolysis, the AAP recommends initiating phototherapy (see below), according to a threshold for serum bilirubin that depends on the infant's age: 15 mg/dL for 25–48 hours; 18 mg/dL for 49–72 hours; and 20 mg/dL for ≥ 72 hours. These values, however, are not very well documented in the literature and cannot be used for infants who are preterm, ill, or have hemolysis. Many clinicians also will use lower values than these, because of the ease of phototherapy and its low risk vs. the risk of kernicterus in the untreated infant. Clinical judgment is usually required for many infants, based on a practitioner's personal experience.

Kernicterus

Essentially, this refers to the neurologic problems that occur when you have yellow sludge dumped on your brain cells. Okay, more scientifically, it is the deposition of unconjugated bilirubin into brain cells—particularly into the basal ganglia. Note: The value at which this occurs varies from infant to infant, and there is no true, absolute, safety level. Even in term newborns, kernicterus can occur with a serum bilirubin level < 25 mg/dL, but it is very rare without some underlying hemolysis or other factor. We do know that the more premature the infant, the more likely he/she is to be affected by hyperbilirubinemia. Bilirubin also can affect other cells. It inhibits mitochondrial enzymes and can cause DNA strand breakage, as well as interfere with DNA synthesis.

What determines if the baby will have kernicterus? It really depends on the concentration of bilirubin in the brain and the duration the brain has been exposed to high concentrations. The presence of hemolysis seems to modify the risk significantly. For example, in an infant with Rh hemolytic disease, a peak serum bilirubin level of 20 mg/dL predicts a poor outcome; but infants with levels higher than this also can be normal! The features are outlined in Table 8-10. An MRI will show good correlation with deposition of bilirubin in the basal ganglion. Long-term effects vary, and many children are clinically healthy later in life. However, boys are much more likely than girls to have long-term effects.

Newer transcutaneous devices that use multiwavelength spectral reflectance correlate very well with serum bilirubin levels in newborns. Also, since CO and bilirubin are produced in the same amounts when heme is broken down, newer devices measure exhaled CO in infants to monitor for increased rates of bilirubin levels.

How to prevent hyperbilirubinemia? By either reducing the bilirubin in the enterohepatic circulation or by inhibiting bilirubin production. Increasing the number of oral feedings in the newborn increases the excretion of bilirubin and reduces the amount of bilirubin in the enterohepatic circulation. No agent for infants has been effective in reducing the bilirubin in the enterohepatic circulation; and, as of yet, no agent is approved for inhibiting bilirubin production. However, early studies with tin-mesoporphyrin are promising.

Treatment of Hyperbilirubinemia

Whom do you treat? (See Table 8-11 and Table 8-12.) Treatment depends on the infant's gestational age, serum bilirubin level, and age of the infant when the level was drawn. Don't memorize these two tables and their values, but be familiar with a general rationale regarding who requires phototherapy or exchange transfusion. The key in the exam question will likely be significant risk factors as mentioned in Table 8-11 and Table 8-12.

The standard treatment is usually phototherapy. Phototherapy produces lumirubin—a water-soluble compound that is the rate-limiting step in elimination of bilirubin by phototherapy. 2 factors determine the rate of lumirubin formation—the wavelength of light and the total dose of light. Remember: Bilirubin is yellow; therefore, it is most likely to absorb blue light (it has a wavelength of 450 nm). However, blue light causes eyestrain and other problems and is rarely used in hospitals. Green light will penetrate the skin more deeply, but fluorescent white light is still the most commonly used light. Dose delivery (remember your physics) is proportional to the power of the light and the distance from the baby. Usually, 8 fluorescent white bulbs are used to deliver 6–12 $\mu W/cm^2$ of

notes

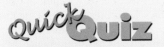

1) Describe the initial workup in an infant with hyperbilirubinemia.

2) What is kernicterus?

3) What will increasing the number of feeds in a newborn do to bilirubin excretion?

4) Describe the treatment approaches for hyperbilirubinemia.

5) What are the complications of exchange transfusion?

6) Describe erythroblastosis fetalis. [Know it well!]

7) True or False: The newborn with erythroblastosis fetalis is likely to be jaundiced at birth. Why or why not?

body-surface area exposed per nanometer of wavelength. Fiberoptic blankets can also be used and provide up to 50 µW/cm^2/nm. Remember: Always shield the baby's eyes. Because of the heat from the lights, there is an increase in insensible water loss; therefore you must monitor the temperature and hydration status of the baby. You can stop phototherapy once the serum bilirubin has been decreased by 4–5 mg/dL. Rebound hyperbilirubinemia, once thought to be common, is now rare in term newborns.

Exchange transfusion is useful when infants have ongoing hemolysis. Here, 1 or 2 central venous catheters are placed, and small amounts of blood are removed and replaced with similar amounts of RBCs mixed with plasma from a compatible donor crossmatched to both the infant and mother. This is done until twice the blood volume has been replaced. Some practitioners recommend infusion of salt-poor albumin (increases the amount of bound bilirubin) before the exchange transfusion to increase the amount of bilirubin removed.

The biggest problems with exchange transfusions are their complications:
- Thrombocytopenia
- Portal vein thrombosis
- NEC
- Electrolyte problems
- Graft-versus-host
- Infections

Table 8-11: Guidelines for Implementing Phototherapy in Hyperbilirubinemia

For infants at low risk (≥ 38 weeks gestation and without risk factors), phototherapy is started at the following total serum bilirubin values:
- 24 hours of age: > 12 mg/dL (205 micromol/L)
- 48 hours of age: > 15 mg/dL (257 micromol/L)
- 72 hours of age: > 18 mg/dL (308 micromol/L)

Infants in this category who have TSB levels 2 to 3 mg/dL (35 to 51 micromol/L) below the recommended levels may be treated with fiberoptic or conventional phototherapy at home.

For infants at medium risk (≥ 38 weeks gestation with risk factors or 35 to 37 6/7 weeks gestation without risk factors), phototherapy is started at the following total serum bilirubin values:
- 24 hours of age: > 10 mg/dL (171 micromol/L)
- 48 hours of age: > 13 mg/dL (222 micromol/L)
- 72 hours of age: > 15 mg/dL (257 micromol/L)

For infants at high risk (35 to 37 6/7 weeks gestation with risk factors), phototherapy is initiated at the following total serum bilirubin values:
- 24 hours of age: > 8 mg/dL (137 micromol/L)
- 48 hours of age: > 11 mg/dL (188 micromol/L)
- 72 hours of age: > 13.5 mg/dL (231 micromol/L)

Table 8-12: Guidelines for Implementing Exchange Transfusion in Hyperbilirubinemia

The following are age-based total serum bilirubin threshold values for exchange transfusion recommended by the AAP based upon gestational age and the presence or absence of risk factors (isoimmune hemolytic disease, glucose-6-phosphate dehydrogenase [G6PD] deficiency, asphyxia, significant lethargy, temperature instability, sepsis, acidosis, or albumin < 3.0 g/dL [if measured]):

For infants at low risk (≥ 38 weeks gestation and without risk factors), exchange transfusion is indicated for the following total serum bilirubin values:
- 24 hours of age: > 19 mg/dL (325 micromol/L)
- 48 hours of age: > 22 mg/dL (376 micromol/L)
- 72 hours of age: > 24 mg/dL (410 micromol/L)
- Any age: ≥ 25 mg/dL (428 micromol/L)

For infants at medium risk (≥ 38 weeks gestation with risk factors or 35 to 37 6/7 weeks gestation without risk factors), exchange transfusion is indicated for the following total serum bilirubin values:
- 24 hours of age: > 16.5 mg/dL (282 micromol/L)
- 48 hours of age: > 19 mg/dL (325 micromol/L)
- ≥ 72 hours of age: > 21 mg/dL (359 micromol/L)

For infants at high risk (35 to 37 6/7 weeks gestation with risk factors), exchange transfusion is indicated for the following total serum bilirubin values:
- 24 hours of age: > 15 mg/dL (257 micromol/L)
- 48 hours of age: > 17 mg/dL (291 micromol/L)
- ≥ 72 hours of age: > 18.5 mg/dL (316 micromol/L)

notes

In infants with other problems besides isolated hyper-bilirubinemia, the complication rate is high. In healthy term infants with hyperbilirubinemia, the complication rate is very low, but it is still advisable to attempt phototherapy first. If phototherapy fails, or if the bilirubin appears that it will reach 25 mg/dL by 48 hours of life and the risk of encephalopathy is high, perform exchange transfusion.

Phenobarbital was used in the past but has fallen out of favor with most experts.

If encephalopathy has already occurred and bilirubin has accumulated in the brain, alkalinize the blood (7.45–7.55 pH) to correct abnormalities in auditory-evoked potentials.

BLOOD DISORDERS IN THE NEWBORN

ERYTHROBLASTOSIS FETALIS

Erythroblastosis fetalis (hemolytic disease of the newborn) occurs when maternal antibodies active against RBC antigens of the infant are passed transplacentally. This leads to increased RBC destruction. > 60 different RBC antigens can induce this, but it is usually associated with the D antigen of the Rh group or with ABO incompatibility.

The Rh antigens are determined genetically by both parents and direct production of a bunch of blood group factors (C, c, D, E, e; there is no "d" antigen, only the "absence of D"). 90% of reactions to Rh antigens are due to D antigen, with the remaining due to C or E. A woman who is D-negative can become sensitized during her pregnancy with a D-positive fetus when fetal RBCs cross the placenta in the second and third trimester, and at delivery. Sensitization is also variable and does not occur in every instance. If the mother continues to have D-positive fetuses, her antibody titers increase and can cause more severe disease in future children. This can be prevented if the mom is given anti-D globulin (RhoGAM) during her third trimester and again at delivery of her D-positive infant. This must be done with each pregnancy! The mother, if not desensitized, will create IgG antibodies against D. These will cross the placenta and cause harm to fetal RBCs. Hemolysis is variable and can be mild to severe. In mild cases, the infant can go to term. In moderate cases, preterm labor is common. In severe hemolysis, intrauterine transfusions may be required.

What happens in the fetus? Once fetal RBCs have maternal antibodies attached to them, they go to the reticuloendothelial system and are hemolyzed. The fetus becomes anemic. At this point, the fetus responds by cranking up erythropoiesis and produces tons of erythroblasts. There can be as many as 40–100,000 erythroblasts/dL. This huge jump in erythropoiesis can deplete the pluripotential hematopoietic stem cells to the point that the WBCs fall to neutropenic levels, and the platelet count also falls dangerously, so the fetus becomes pancytopenic.

You'd think with all this hemolysis, the baby would be born yellow, right? Well, the unconjugated bilirubin from the fetus crosses the placenta and then is conjugated by the mother and eliminated, so the baby at birth is usually not jaundiced in appearance, but will become so quickly. Additionally, the cranking up of erythropoiesis will cause the spleen and liver to become dramatically enlarged as they become the sites for RBC precursor production. Splenic rupture at delivery is not uncommon. If the liver is damaged from all of this increased workload, conjugated hyperbilirubinemia may be present at birth.

Also note: Elevated plasma hemoglobin from hemolysis will interfere with insulin function. This will result in hyperinsulinemia and the development of pancreatic islet cell hyperplasia. Once delivery occurs, the baby can become severely hypoglycemic. As the anemia worsens, blood flow increases to vital organs to compensate for the lack of oxygen to these tissues. This process can result in increased fluid load with development of ascites, pleural effusions, and generalized fetal edema.

notes

MedStudy®

4th Edition

Pediatrics Board Review Core Curriculum

Genetics

Authored by J. Thomas Cross, Jr., MD, MPH, FAAP, and Robert A. Hannaman, MD

Many thanks to

Kim Keppler-Noreuil, MD
Clinical Professor of Pediatrics
Program Director of Medical Genetics Residency
Clinical Director of the Iowa Registry of Congenital and Inherited Disorders
Division of Medical Genetics
The University of Iowa Children's Hospital
Iowa City, IA

Genetics Advisor

Table of Contents

Genetics

KEY DEFINITIONS IN GENETIC DISORDERS 9-1
SINGLE GENE DISORDERS
  CLASSIC MENDELIAN INHERITANCE............................... 9-1
    AUTOSOMAL DOMINANT DISORDERS.............................. 9-1
    AUTOSOMAL RECESSIVE DISORDERS 9-2
    X-LINKED DISORDERS... 9-3
    ATYPICAL PATTERNS OF INHERITANCE......................... 9-4
      Mendelian vs. Atypical Inheritance 9-4
      Genomic Imprinting 9-4
      Uniparental Disomy.. 9-4
      Mitochondrial Disorders...................................... 9-4
      Trinucleotide Repeat Diseases 9-5
MULTIFACTORIAL INHERITANCE.................................... 9-6
TWINS FACTS 9-6
RISKS OF GENETIC DISEASE 9-6
TRISOMY SYNDROMES 9-7
  TRISOMY 21 (DOWN SYNDROME) 9-7
    Incidence/Screening 9-7
    Presentation 9-7
    Heart Defects in Down Syndrome 9-8
    GI Defects in Down Syndrome 9-8
    Ocular Problems 9-8
    Developmental Disorders 9-8
    Other Problems of Down Syndrome in Childhood............ 9-8
    Problems of Older Patients with Down Syndrome 9-8
    Anticipatory Guidance for Children with Down Syndrome ... 9-8
    Future Risk of Sibling with Down Syndrome.................. 9-8
  TRISOMY 18 (EDWARDS SYNDROME)............................ 9-9
  TRISOMY 13 (PATAU SYNDROME) 9-9
  MOSAIC TRISOMY 8.. 9-9
DELETION SYNDROMES.. 9-10
  OVERVIEW 9-10
  4p- (WOLF-HIRSCHHORN SYNDROME)........................... 9-10
  5p- (CRI-DU-CHAT SYNDROME) 9-10
  18q- (De GROUCHY SYNDROME) 9-10
  OTHER DELETIONS 9-10
MICRODELETION OR CONTIGUOUS GENE SYNDROMES... 9-11
  OVERVIEW 9-11
  15q11-13 (ANGELMAN
    AND PRADER-WILLI SYNDROMES)............................ 9-11
    Maternal vs. Paternal... 9-11
    Maternally Derived 15q11-13 (Angelman Syndrome) 9-11
    Paternally Derived 15q11-13 (Prader-Willi Syndrome) 9-11
  7q11.23- (WILLIAMS SYNDROME) 9-12
  11p13- (WAGR SYNDROME) 9-12
  20p12- (ALAGILLE SYNDROME)................................... 9-12
  22q11.2- (VELOCARDIOFACIAL/
    DiGEORGE SYNDROME) 9-12
SEX CHROMOSOME ABNORMALITIES 9-13
  INCIDENCE 9-13
  47,XXY (KLINEFELTER SYNDROME) 9-13
  OTHER EXTRA X CHROMOSOME SYNDROMES................. 9-13
  47,XYY MALE 9-13
  45,X (TURNER SYNDROME)....................................... 9-13
CHROMOSOMAL INSTABILITY SYNDROMES 9-14
ANOMALIES OF THE HEAD 9-14
  CLEFT LIP / PALATE DISORDERS 9-14
    Pierre-Robin Sequence 9-14
    Amniotic Band Sequence 9-14
  HEMIFACIAL MICROSOMIA 9-14

Findings.. 9-14
  Goldenhar Syndrome 9-15
OTHER FACIAL ANOMALY SYNDROMES 9-15
  Branchio-Oto-Renal (BOR) Syndrome 9-15
  Treacher-Collins Syndrome
    (Mandibulofacial Dysostosis Type 1) 9-15
CRANIOSYNOSTOSIS.. 9-15
PLAGIOCEPHALY (Positional Flattening of the Skull) 9-15
SKELETAL DYSPLASIAS.. 9-16
  ACHONDROPLASIA... 9-16
  THANATOPHORIC DYSPLASIAS 9-16
CARTILAGE ANOMALIES 9-16
  OSTEOGENESIS IMPERFECTA 9-16
    All Types 9-16
    Osteogenesis Imperfecta Type I................................ 9-16
    Osteogenesis Imperfecta Type II............................... 9-16
    Osteogenesis Imperfecta Type III.............................. 9-17
    Osteogenesis Imperfecta Type IV.............................. 9-17
CONNECTIVE TISSUE DYSPLASIAS................................. 9-17
  MARFAN SYNDROME.. 9-17
  EHLERS-DANLOS SYNDROMES 9-18
NEUROCUTANEOUS DISEASES 9-19
  NEUROFIBROMATOSIS TYPE 1 9-19
  NEUROFIBROMATOSIS TYPE 2 9-19
  TUBEROUS SCLEROSIS 9-20
CANCER GENETIC SYNDROMES 9-20
  von HIPPEL-LINDAU SYNDROME 9-20
  THE *PTEN* HAMARTOMA TUMOR SYNDROME............... 9-21
  TWO-HIT ORIGIN OF CANCER 9-21
  TERATOGENS 9-21
    Thalidomide 9-21
    Carbamazepine... 9-21
    Methotrexate 9-21
    ACE Inhibitors 9-21
    Diethylstilbestrol (DES) 9-21
    Lithium.. 9-22
    Phenytoin 9-22
    Retinoic Acid 9-22
    Streptomycin 9-22
    Tetracycline... 9-22
    Valproic Acid 9-22
    Warfarin 9-22
  MATERNAL EXPOSURES AND ABUSES 9-22
    Alcohol.. 9-22
    Cigarette Smoking 9-22
    Cocaine 9-23
    Mercury (Fish Ingestion) 9-23
  MATERNAL DISEASES 9-23
    Diabetes Mellitus 9-23
    Hypertension 9-23
    Hyperthermia (Hot Tub Users and High Maternal Fever).... 9-23
    Systemic Lupus Erythematosus (SLE)......................... 9-23
  MATERNAL INFECTIONS 9-23
    Note 9-23
    Human Parvovirus B19 (Fifth Disease) 9-23
    Varicella.. 9-23
    Rubella 9-23
    Cytomegalovirus (CMV)....................................... 9-23
    Toxoplasmosis 9-23
    Syphilis 9-23

At first glance, you would think that congenital, hereditary, and familial all mean the same thing. But they don't. Take this example: Trisomy 21, infection with rubella, and amniotic bands are all congenital conditions. Congenital refers to a condition or anomaly present at birth. Of the three, though, only trisomy 21 is a genetic condition, and none of these is hereditary. Hereditary refers to conditions that can be transmitted from parent to offspring. All hereditary conditions are genetic but not all genetic conditions are hereditary, as in the example of trisomy 21. (Does this sound like college philosophy 101?) Familial refers to conditions that "cluster" in families and can include nongenetic (streptococcal infections, chicken pox), as well as genetic conditions. And to add more philosophy 101, all hereditary conditions are familial, but not all genetic conditions are familial (trisomy 21). Genotype refers to the genetic constitution or different forms of a gene (alleles) at a given locus. Phenotype refers to observed expression (physical, biochemical, or physiological findings) of the genotype or gene mutation.

Penetrance refers to the ability of a known disease-causing genotype to be expressed or to exhibit the disease phenotype. Reduced or incomplete penetrance means that the gene is not expressed 100% of the time. The example in the texts (and probably on the Board exam) is retinoblastoma. We know from population studies that about 10% who have an autosomal dominant gene mutation causing retinoblastoma do not develop retinoblastoma. Thus, the penetrance for this condition is 90%.

Variable expressivity refers to individuals who have the same genetic condition (and sometimes even the exact same genotype) but present with different phenotypes. For example, Treacher-Collins syndrome is an autosomal dominant, craniofacial malformation syndrome; within the same family, some children may have cleft palate while others do not.

Pleiotropic refers to genes that produce many effects. An example of this is Marfan syndrome, which can affect the eye, cardiovascular system, and skeletal system.

Heterozygous refers to 2 different alleles at a locus on a pair of homologous chromosomes, while homozygous refers to identical alleles at a particular gene locus. A mutation is the term used to describe a change in the DNA code.

Autosome refers to all chromosomes except the X or Y chromosome. There are 22 autosomes, numbers 1–22, and 2 sex chromosomes, X and Y. The majority of the population has a total of 46 chromosomes, 2 copies of each autosome and either XX or XY to determine the sex of the person. When there are extra or missing autosomes or sex chromosomes, this abnormality is referred to as aneuploidy.

Anomaly in clinical genetics terminology refers to a structural birth defect or congenital malformation. Multiple anomalies may form recognized patterns of malformation known as syndrome, sequence, association, complex, or phenotype.

Phenotype: A composite of features that may be due to multiple causes. Example: Pena-Shokeir phenotype. Complex: anoma-lies of several different structures that lie together in the same local body region during embryonic development (developmental field). Example: Limb-body wall complex. Syndrome: A recognizable pattern of structural defects, often with a predictable natural history that can be identified amongst several patients. Example: Cornelia de Lange syndrome, Williams syndrome. Sequence: A pattern of multiple anomalies that results from a single identifiable event in development. Example: Pierre-Robin sequence.

SINGLE GENE DISORDERS CLASSIC MENDELIAN INHERITANCE

AUTOSOMAL DOMINANT DISORDERS

Autosomal dominant (AD) disorders are phenotypically expressed with only 1 copy of an altered allele. (See Figure 9-1.) AD disorders occur more commonly than the other single gene disorders, but each individual disorder is still rare; therefore it would be unusual, based just on statistical odds, for two people with the same AD disorder to mate. A heterozygous parent has a 50% chance of passing the disorder to his/her children.

When given a pedigree on the test to determine if AD is the mode of transmission, look for:
- Both sexes are equally affected.
- Both sexes can transmit to offspring.
- No generation is skipped (unless the trait is subtle or not completely expressed; then you may not notice it in that generation).
- Every affected child has a parent with the disorder (except if this is a new gene mutation; then this child's offspring will have a 50% risk of inheriting this gene mutation.
- You see father-to-son transmission (this excludes all X-linked and mitochondrial transmissions).

"Spontaneous" mutations can occur, and are important, in AD disorders; e.g., neurofibromatosis Type 1, where ~ 60% of cases are due to new dominant mutations. Some factors increase the risk of new dominant mutations, one being older paternal age (because of DNA copy errors in the spermatocytes). For example, the older the father, the more likely he is to have a child with achondroplasia or Marfan syndrome.

One "fly in the ointment" is germline mosaicism. Consider this

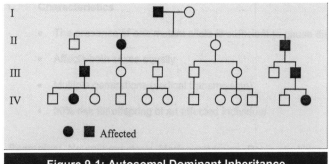

Figure 9-1: Autosomal Dominant Inheritance

scenario when an AD disorder arises from a germline mutation: The appearance of an autosomal dominant (AD) trait—one affected child, unaffected parents, and no other affected family members. The parent carries the gene mutation in their gonadal tissue and germline cells, but not in the somatic cells—and does not show signs of the disease; therefore, their offspring are at an increased risk (~ 5–10%) to inherit this condition. It is suspected when a "normal" parent has more than one child affected with an autosomal dominant or X-linked condition. Note: Germline mosaicism also occurs in X-linked inherited disorders or traits.

AUTOSOMAL RECESSIVE DISORDERS

Autosomal recessive (AR) disorders require 2 copies of an altered allele to produce a disease phenotype. (See Figure 9-2.) AR disorders are less common than AD disorders in most populations, but heterozygote carriers (having only 1 altered allele) are much more common in the general population.

Keys on the pedigree for AR disorders:
- Look for disorders in one or more siblings, but not in other generations.
- Males and females are equally affected.
- Males and females can each transmit the altered allele.
- The risk for 2 heterozygotes to have an affected offspring is 1/4. (However, 2 heterozygotes also can have offspring who are all affected or all unaffected!)
- Consanguinity increases the risk of having an offspring with an AR disorder (see Figure 9-3).

Sometimes, the Board exam will ask you to calculate probabilities or population frequencies for various diseases. Hopefully, they won't, but here is how to do some complicated calculations, just in case. Cystic fibrosis (CF) is a disorder that is commonly used as an example for AR inheritance. CF has an incidence of ~ 1/1,600, with a relatively high carrier frequency in the general Caucasian population: ~ 1/20. Therefore, the general population risk for a Caucasian couple to have a child with CF would be 1/20 x 1/20 x 1/4 (AR risk to have an affected child) = 1/1,600.

Let's say we have an allele that is black hair (B) and one that is white hair (b), that "B" is an AD trait such that any "B" in a genotype will confer black hair, and that the only way to have white hair is to have genotype bb.

Then let's say that at a 2-allele locus, the frequency "p" of the dominant allele, "B," is 0.80. This means that 80% of the sperm cells and 80% of the egg cells in a population have allele "B." The sum of the 2 possible allele frequencies must equal 1. Therefore, the frequency "q" of the recessive allele, "b," is $1 - p = q$, or $1 - 0.8 = 0.2$.

So, using this equation, the chance that a sperm containing the dominant allele "B" unites with an egg carrying the dominant allele "B" is $p \times p = 0.8 \times 0.8 = 0.64$. And the probability of producing an offspring with both recessive genes or having the "bb" genotype is $q \times q = 0.2 \times 0.2 = 0.04$.

Two things can happen to produce a heterozygote: 1) a sperm with "B" can unite with an egg carrying "b", or 2) a sperm carrying "b" can unite with an egg carrying "B." So, the frequency with which this occurs is the sum of the product of each possibility. $(p \times q) + (p \times q) = 2 (p \times q) = 2 (0.8 \times 0.2) = 0.32$.

Putting it all together, what is the frequency of white hair in the community? It is 0.04 or 4%. Note that the frequencies have to add up to 1: $0.64 (BB) + 0.32 (Bb \text{ or } bB) + 0.04 (bb) = 1$

Now, this is different from me asking: What is the probability of two carriers (heterozygotes) producing a child with white hair, a child who is heterozygous, and a child who is homozygous for black hair?

Here, we know that mom is Bb and dad is Bb. Thus, the egg mom contributes to the baby will be either a B egg or a b egg, and dad's sperm will be either a B sperm or a b sperm.

So the chance that junior will be white-haired (bb) is (the chance that dad's sperm is b) x (the chance that mom's egg is b) which is (1/2) x (1/2) = 1/4 ... or a 25% chance.

If mom and dad already have 2 children with white hair (bb), what is the chance that the next baby will have white hair (bb)? Exactly the same: 1/4 or 25%—the mom's egg and the dad's sperm for making this new baby don't have any recollection of what happened in the past, and they don't have a tote board saying, "Wow, we've already had 2 white-haired babies, so the chance we'll have another white-haired baby again is pretty low."

Now, this is different from asking before they have any children: "What is the chance that if they have 3 kids, all 3 will have white hair?"

That would be 1/4 x 1/4 x 1/4 = 1/64.

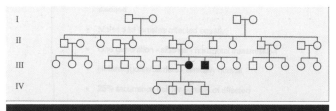

Figure 9-2: Autosomal Recessive Inheritance

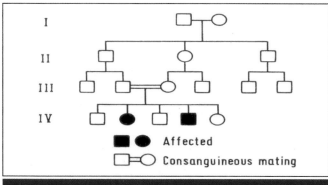

Figure 9-3: AR with Consanguinity

notes

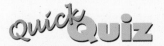

1) Define the terms hereditary, familial, variable expressivity, heterozygous, homozygous, genotype, and phenotype.

2) Know how to differentiate on a pedigree: autosomal dominant, autosomal recessive, and X-linked disorders.

3) What is germline mosaicism?

4) Which form of classic Mendelian inheritance does not have male-to-male transmission?

5) Which form of classic Mendelian inheritance has a father passing the disease allele to all of his daughters and none of his sons?

X-LINKED DISORDERS

The X chromosome is twice as large as the Y chromosome and has thousands of genes compared to the poor Y, which has ~ 25 identified genes localized to it, including one especially important gene (*SRY* gene, sex-determining region Y). Many well-known pediatric diseases are caused by mutations in genes on the X-chromosome, including:

• hemophilia A,
• Duchenne and Becker muscular dystrophy, and
• red-green color blindness.

Over 100 different phenotypes associated with mental retardation have been mapped to the X chromosome (for example, fragile X syndrome).

So, you are wondering: "Gee, females have 2 X copies and males have only 1 X copy, so females must have a lot more X-linked gene products." (Okay, maybe you weren't wondering that.) However, this is not the case because of what we call "dosage compensation," which is produced by the inactivation of one of the X chromosomes early in female embryonic life. It usually begins about 2 weeks after fertilization. This is a random process, so the inactivated X chromosome (*in each cell*) could come from either the mother or the father. So, somatic cells in the female embryo will each have about a 50% chance of having an active X from the mom and 50% from the dad. This further means that females will have 2 populations of cells known as somatic mosaicism. This becomes evident if the maternally and paternally derived X chromosomes produce different products! An example occurs in women who are carriers for X-linked ocular albinism; they will have patches of pigmented and nonpigmented cells that correspond to whether the cells have the disease-bearing X chromosome (nonpigmented) or the normal X chromosome (pigmented).

In some cases, the "extra" X chromosome is not completely inactivated, and genes in several regions continue to be transcribed from the inactivated X chromosome. So, females can be homozygous for a disease allele at a given locus, heterozygous for one disease allele and one normal allele, or homozygous for a normal allele at a locus. Males have only one X chromosome and are considered "hemizygous" for an allele at a locus on the X chromosome. Thus, if a male inherits an X-linked recessive allele for a disease, he will be affected. On the other hand, an X-linked dominant disease can cause disease in either males or females, because the presence of only one copy of an altered allele is sufficient for disease to occur.

For males with X-linked recessive disorders, the frequency of the disease in males = the frequency of the gene, q. This is because all males with the altered gene have the disease condition. For females, the frequency of the gene condition will be $q \times q$, because they need both alleles to express the disease.

For example, let's say that being a red smurf (as opposed to the normal blue) is X-linked recessive, and that the prevalence in males is about 1/5,000 ($q = .0002$). Thus, you will see affected females in $q \times q = .0002 \times .0002 = 0.00000004$—or 1/25,000,000 females.

Here, I'm including an example disorder having X-linked inheritance with their clinical descriptions: Duchenne muscular dystrophy (more on this later as well). This is an important disorder that you should know—and it appears very frequently in Board questions.

Duchenne muscular dystrophy commonly presents with:

• progressive muscle weakness,
• calf hypertrophy, and
• Gowers sign at ~ 2 years of age.

Other findings: cardiomyopathy and 33% of patients have cognitive delays.

Keys to remember concerning X-linked recessive pedigrees (see Figure 9-4):

• Only females can transmit the disease to their sons; there is never male-to-male transmission.
• If a generation has only females, the disease will appear to have "skipped" that generation.
• An affected father transmits the disease allele to all his daughters (the daughters are obligate carriers, but usually unaffected).
• Carrier females have a 50% chance of transmitting the disease to their sons.

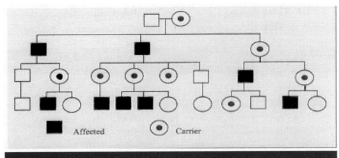

Figure 9-4: X-linked Recessive Inheritance

notes

Now, why do some female "carriers" have some or all manifestations of an X-linked recessive disorder? There are 3 possibilities:

1) Remember: Inactivation of the X chromosome is a random process within each cell. Sometimes, a much higher proportion of X chromosomes with a normal allele are inactivated than X chromosomes that carry a disease allele. These girls are "manifesting heterozygotes" and usually have a milder form of the condition. A common example is seen in hemophilia A, where 5% of women who carry one of the alleles for hemophilia A will have factor VIII levels low enough to exhibit mild forms of the disease.

2) Some girls have only a single X chromosome (Turner syndrome).

Deletions or rearrangements in an X chromosome and another non-X chromosome (autosome) can result in affected females, which is rare.

ATYPICAL PATTERNS OF INHERITANCE

Mendelian vs. Atypical Inheritance

Some single gene disorders do not follow the autosomal dominant, autosomal recessive, or X-linked recessive patterns of inheritance (classic Mendelian inheritance). In classic Mendelian inheritance, the expression of the disease is independent of the parent with the causative allele. The following situations are examples of when it does matter from which parent the child gets the allele.

Genomic Imprinting

Genomic (genetic) imprinting refers to differences in gene expression, depending on whether the disease allele is inherited from the mother or the father. For example, when deletion of a 2–4 Mb portion of chromosome 15 is inherited from the father, the child is born with Prader-Willi syndrome. This syndrome presents with severe hypotonia, obesity, small hands and feet, and mental retardation. Thus, the deletion of all paternally active genes from this part of the chromosome results in Prader-Willi syndrome. When the deletion is inherited from the mother, the child is born with Angelman syndrome. Children with Angelman syndrome may appear normal at birth, but by 6–12 months of age usually develop seizures, mental retardation, microcephaly, ataxia, hand-flapping behaviors, and a characteristic "puppet-like" gait. (This is why children with Angelman syndrome in the past were identified by the phrase "the happy puppet"; today, this is considered inappropriate and derogatory, as are many similar "older terms." However, I mention it because it may help you remember the syndrome for the test—but, in the real world, please never use this term!) The deletion of all of the maternally active genes from this part of the chromosome results in Angelman syndrome.

But it isn't so simple. This explains only 70% of the cases of Angelman and Prader-Willi syndromes, which leads us to ask: what about the other 30%?

Uniparental Disomy

Uniparental disomy occurs if both copies of a chromosome—in a part of, or the whole chromosome—are from only one parent. Thus, considering our case above, if a child inherits both copies of maternal chromosome 15, the child lacks the paternally active genes and develops Prader-Willi syndrome. On the other hand, if the child gets both copies from the dad, the child lacks maternally active genes and develops Angelman syndrome. Uniparental disomy arises because of nondisjunction of chromosomes during meiosis in the gametes, which results in trisomy (with subsequent loss of 1 chromosome), or in monosomy (with subsequent duplication of the chromosome). In both cases, the resulting disomic cell line then has 2 chromosomes originating from only 1 parent. Another condition, which can be caused by uniparental disomy or imprinting defects, is Beckwith-Wiedemann syndrome (refer to Table 9-6 at the back of this section).

Mitochondrial Disorders

Mitochondria have the only genetic material outside of the nucleus. However, the mitochondrial genome is haploid (contains only 1 copy of each gene), not diploid like the nucleus. Mitochondrial inheritance is unique because the ovum, not the sperm, transmits all of the mitochondria to their zygote; therefore, a mother carrying a mitochondrial DNA (mtDNA) mutation will pass it on to all her offspring, whereas the father carrying the mutation passes it to none, the majority of times (see Figure 9-5). At cell division, mtDNA replicate and randomly separate in the daughter cells, resulting in different proportions of mitochondria carrying normal and mutant (disease-causing) mtDNA. Heteroplasmy refers to the variable proportion of mutant and normal mtDNA within a cell or tissue. Homoplasmy refers to the state in which all mtDNA are identical.

If a mutation occurs in one copy of mtDNA, the other copy will be unaffected, which results in heteroplasmy—the state of having 2 different mtDNA within a mitochondrion. Mutant mtDNA results in cell death and tissue/organ deterioration. Common presentations for mitochondrial disorders include metabolic encephalopathy, cardiac failure, liver failure, and/or lactic acidosis. mtDNA disorders are not common but account for many cerebrovascular accidents, deafness, and diabetes in children.

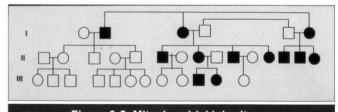

Figure 9-5: Mitochondrial Inheritance

notes   Beckwith-Wiedemann also a d/o of genomic imprinting/uniparental disomy
                    chromo 11

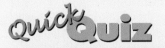
A few disorders are caused by mutations in the mitochondrial genome:
- Myoclonic epilepsy and red-ragged fibers (MERRF) is associated with progressive myoclonic epilepsy, myopathy, dementia, and hearing loss.
- Mitochondrial encephalopathy, with stroke-like episodes, and lactic acidosis (MELAS) present anytime between the ages of toddler and adolescent.
- Leigh disease presents with basal ganglia defects, hypotonia, and optic atrophy in infancy or early childhood.
- Kearns-Sayre syndrome presents with ophthalmoplegia, retinitis pigmentosa, myopathy, and cardiac conduction defects.
- Pearson syndrome presents with anemia, neutropenia, pancreatic dysfunction, and myopathy in infants.

Trinucleotide Repeat Diseases

Triplet is defined as a series of 3 bases in DNA or RNA coding for a specific amino acid. Triplet repeats are normally stably transmitted. Expansion of triplet repeat sequences is unstable and is responsible for a number of diseases.

Fragile X syndrome, the most common inherited mental retardation syndrome, occurs in 1/1,650 males. Originally, a "fragile site" on chromosome Xq27.3 was identified by cytogenetic analysis in a folate-deficient media. It is an X-linked inheritance; however, it exhibited features not usually seen with X-linked inheritance:
- 30% of carrier females have a similar clinical phenotype to that of affected males.
- A normal male could transmit the gene to his daughters, who subsequently would have a 50% risk of having an affected male.

The etiology: caused by an unstable CGG (cytosine-guanine-guanine) repeat in the 5′ untranslated region of the fragile X mental retardation (FMR1) gene on the X chromosome.
- Normal = 6 to 50 repeats
- Premutation = 55 to 200 repeats
- Full mutation = > 200 repeats

Full mutation blocks transcription and is associated with methylation of the CpG (cytosine and guanine separated by a phosphate) island.

Common clinical findings:
- Mental retardation
- Large head
- Long face with large ears
- Large hands and feet
- Macroorchidism
- Hyperextensible joints

Premutation carriers (55 to 200 CGG repeats):
- Previously regarded as being clinically uninvolved
- Presently 3 distinct clinical disorders
- Mild cognitive and/or behavioral deficits on the fragile X–spectrum
- Premature ovarian failure
- Neurodegenerative disorder of older adult carriers, fragile X–associated tremor/ataxia syndrome (FXTAS)

Females with premutation range (> 100 CGG repeats):
- Increased risk of emotional problems: mild form of anxiety and perseverative thinking, depression, interpersonal sensitivity
- Premature ovarian failure in ~ 20%
- Ovarian dysfunction in 20%
- Mild decrease in FMR1 protein

FXTAS (fragile X–associated tremor/ataxia syndrome):
- Less common in females
- Mostly in male carriers, usually > 50 years of age for onset
- > 30% of male carriers develop symptoms
- Significant variability in progression of symptoms
- Clinical criteria: intention tremor and gait ataxia, parkinsonism

Myotonic dystrophy is another triplet repeat disease with these clinical features:
- Autosomal dominant, with variable age of onset and variable severity.
- Myotonia with progressive weakness and wasting; involvement of facial and jaw muscles (ptosis, atrophy of sternocleidomastoid muscles); myotonia on grip testing.
- Other involved organ systems: eye: cataract; endocrine: testicular atrophy, diabetes mellitus; brain: mental retardation; skin: premature balding in males.
- Congenital myotonic dystrophy: results in marked hypotonia, mental retardation (60–70%), neonatal respiratory distress, feeding difficulties, talipes, and may cause neonatal death.
- Etiology: mutation affecting the CTG (cytosine-thymine-guanine) repeat in the 3′ untranslated region of the myotonin kinase gene on chromosome 19. Normally 5–35 repeats; affected individuals with mutations ≥ 50 to several thousand repeats.
- Severity varies with the number of repeats and anticipation.
- Parent of origin effect: The most severely affected babies inherit their trinucleotide repeat expansion from the mother.

notes

MULTIFACTORIAL INHERITANCE

Most genetic disorders are due to multiple genetic and environmental factors, not to a "single gene" model. Multifactorial inheritance is the most common cause of isolated major anomalies observed in the newborn. Examples include neural tube defects, heart defects, schizophrenia, hyperlipidemia, cleft palate, and clubfoot. Many of these are present at birth but some, such as DM and autism, may not present for many years. As a general rule, empiric risks of recurrence for most isolated major anomalies are typically in the range of 2–6%.

In general, a multifactorial disease occurs when enough "bad" factors "overcome" the good factors. Some refer to these "bad" factors as "liability" factors. In other words, enough liability factors must be present to exceed a threshold to result in the disease. For some diseases, this threshold is different depending on the gender.

A good example is pyloric stenosis. Pyloric stenosis normally occurs in about 1/1,200 females and about 1/300 males. This indicates that the "threshold" for this disease is much higher in females than males. Or, in other words, for a female to get pyloric stenosis, she'd have to have an unusually high number of "liability" factors present, especially compared to the case for a male. So, when a female does in fact get pyloric stenosis, it means she has more of these "bad" factors, and the consequence is that her offspring are much more likely to have this disorder—even more likely than the offspring of an affected male (who presumably would have pyloric stenosis with fewer liability factors present in the first place). Knowing this, let's say you have a woman with a history of pyloric stenosis as a child. Are her boys or her girls more likely to be affected? Boys! Why? Because it takes fewer liability factors—"fewer hoops to jump through"—for males to develop the disease. When the mom is transmitting enough of these factors (remember, we said this is a mother with a history of pyloric stenosis), her son is more likely than her daughter to reach the threshold.

Keys to recognize multifactorial inheritance:
- Recurrence risk increases as the number of affected individuals in the family increases; e.g., the recurrence risk of a disorder is estimated at 2% if one sibling has the disorder, but increases to 12% if 2 siblings have the disorder. Remember: The subsequent risk is the same for single gene disorders; the genetic roulette wheel doesn't remember what has previously occurred.
- The recurrence risk is higher if the affected individual is a member of the less commonly affected sex. See the pyloric stenosis scenario above. This also holds true for infantile autism, where males are 4x more likely than females to be affected. But if a girl in the family has autism, it is twice as likely to recur in a sibling than if a boy is the one with the autism.
- Recurrence risk is higher if the affected individual has a more severe form/case.

- The recurrence risk drops dramatically as the degree of relationship decreases from the affected individual and his/her relatives. For example, if a woman has clubfoot, her 1st degree relative has ~ 2.5% risk of clubfoot, but this drops to 0.5% for a 2nd degree relative, and to 0.2% for a 3rd degree relative. (The general population has a risk of 0.1 %.)
- Recurrence risk correlates with the prevalence in the general population. In single gene disorders, the recurrence risk is independent of the general population: If you have one parent who is heterozygous for a very rare AD disorder and the other parent is unaffected, the risk is 50% that their child will get the disorder. For many multifactorial diseases, the population prevalence p will give a risk of $\sqrt{p}$ for siblings of that affected child.
- Folic acid supplementation both prior to and through early pregnancy has been proven to prevent neural tube defects and possibly reduce the risk of other birth defects.

TWINS FACTS

Remember: There are monozygotic (identical) and dizygotic (fraternal) twins. Monozygotic twins share 100% of their genes! Dizygotic twins are caused by the fertilization of two egg cells by two different sperm cells, and, therefore, they share 50% of their genes; so they are genetically similar to their other siblings, but they just happen to share the same uterus.

Over time, we have learned that a trait strongly influenced by genes shows greater similarity in monozygotic than in dizygotic twins.

Most believe that some traits are strongly influenced by genes, and therefore rates (of trait concordance) between monozygotic and dizygotic twins can be quite varied, as indeed they are in the following:
- Autism (60% concordance in monozygotic twins vs. 0% in dizygotic twins)
- Cleft lip/palate (38% vs. 8%)
- Clubfoot (32% vs. 3%)
- Spina bifida (72% vs. 33%)

RISKS OF GENETIC DISEASE

You will encounter many parents concerned about genetic diseases and specific risks for their particular child. Once a child is born with an abnormality, many parents want to know if this is "genetic" and, therefore, "could this happen again?" Also, on the Board exam, you may be asked to decide if a disorder has a risk of being genetic or not.

Clues that a genetic disorder is likely:
- Previous family history of genetic disorder
- Positive neonatal screen
- Congenital anomalies
- Developmental abnormalities

notes

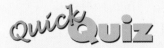

1) What are some of the factors in recognizing that multifactorial inheritance has occurred?

2) Are dizygotic twins more likely, less likely, or equally likely to have genetic traits similar to those of an older sibling?

3) Name 4 diseases or abnormalities that are much more common in monozygotic than dizygotic twins.

4) What is the genetic abnormality in trisomy 21?

5) What is the current theory for the etiology of trisomy 21?

6) What is the only factor shown to increase the risk of trisomy 21?

7) What screening tests may indicate an increased risk of trisomy 21?

8) What are some of the classic physical findings in children with trisomy 21?

- Neurologic disorders
- Death *in utero* or soon after birth
- Growth abnormalities
- Multiorgan dysfunction

Indications for chromosomal analysis:
- Multiple birth defects
- Developmental delay and/or mental retardation
- Growth abnormalities (e.g., short stature)
- Abnormal sexual development
- Recurrent miscarriages

TRISOMY SYNDROMES
TRISOMY 21 (DOWN SYNDROME)

Incidence/Screening

Trisomy 21 is the most common autosomal chromosome trisomy in humans, occurring in 1/800 live births. The incidence in conceptions is more than 2x the incidence at birth, because > 50% of the conceptions abort during early pregnancy. Approximately 94% of those with Down syndrome have 3 copies of the whole chromosome 21 (see Figure 9-6); around 3% will have only part of the long arm due to translocations with chromosomes 14, 15, or 13; and the remaining 3% will have mosaicism.

The etiology of trisomy 21 is the "extra" copy of chromosome 21 and is thought to be due to nondisjunction during meiosis. The only factor shown to increase the risk of having a child with Down syndrome is increasing maternal age. No environmental factors have been implicated.

Screening in women under the age of 35 years can include looking for an abnormal maternal serum screen study, consisting of low maternal serum α-fetoprotein, low unconjugated estriol, elevated hCG, and elevated inhibin levels, all of which may indicate increased risk of a fetus with Down syndrome.

Presentation

Down syndrome presents with a classic phenotypic pattern, but, if taken singly, many of the findings are minor anomalies or nonspecific. You need the "whole picture" to make an accurate diagnosis.

Most commonly found:
- Hypotonia
- Small ears
- Mental retardation

More specific to Down syndrome:
- Brachydactyly: Short, broad fingers and toes (Especially note the broad space between the 1st and 2nd toes! See Figure 9-7.)
- Absent-to-very-small nipple buds (also seen in other disorders)
- Central placement of the posterior hair whorl (also seen in other disorders)

Common in Down syndrome, but nonspecific:
- Microcephaly
- Up-slanted palpebral fissures
- Flat midface
- Full cheeks
- Epicanthal folds
- Single transverse crease (see Figure 9-8)
- Speckled irises (Brushfield spots)
- High-arched palate
- Hypoplasia of the middle phalanx of 5th finger/clinodactyly

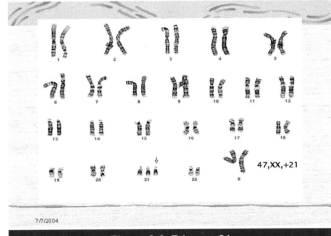

47,XX,+21

7/7/2004

Figure 9-6: Trisomy 21

notes
↓ AFP
↓ estriol
↑ HCG
↑ inhibin

Heart Defects in Down Syndrome

Heart defects are fairly common, occurring in nearly 50% of patients. 1/3 of these are AV canal defects, and 1/3 are VSDs. The other 1/3 have ASDs of the secundum variety and tetralogy of Fallot. Remember that AV canal defects frequently do not have an associated murmur. Since ~ 50% of children with Down syndrome have congenital heart defects, echocardiogram is mandatory for all children with suspected Down syndrome.

GI Defects in Down Syndrome

Duodenal atresia and Hirschsprung disease occur in about 5% of infants with Down syndrome. Look for the classic double-bubble sign, indicating duodenal atresia on abdominal x-rays (see the Gastroenterology & Nutrition section). Most patients will present clinically, and you will not need biopsy or further GI evaluations unless symptoms develop.

Ocular Problems

Congenital cataracts occur in about 5%, but other problems, such as strabismus and refractive errors, are very common; so ensure that careful, routine ophthalmologic evaluations take place.

Developmental Disorders

Children with Down syndrome have developmental delay, with mean IQ scores ranging from 20 to 50; however, social performance is beyond that expected for the mental age. Almost all children learn to walk and communicate, and most progress at a steady but slower pace than usual. Encourage early intervention programs to accelerate milestones in the early years.

Other Problems of Down Syndrome in Childhood

Other problems in childhood can include hypothyroidism, atlantoaxial instability, and leukemia (particularly ALL). Do thyroid function studies at 3, 6, and 12 months, and then annually. Also order C-spine x-rays at ~ 3 years of age, to monitor for atlantoaxial instability.

Problems of Older Patients with Down Syndrome

These problems occur later in life, sometimes in the 20s–40s, but since many pediatricians remain the "physician" for some of these children, you must vigilantly look for these long-term complications:
- DM
- Thyroid disorders (both hypo- and hyperthyroidism)
- Atlantoaxial subluxation
- Cataracts
- Leukemia
- Seizures
- Cognitive dysfunction (during the 40s)
- Dementia or early-onset Alzheimer disease

Anticipatory Guidance for Children with Down Syndrome

- All routine immunizations
- Cardiac evaluation with echocardiogram in the newborn period
- Ophthalmology evaluation before 6 months of age
- Hearing evaluation by 6 months of age
- Thyroid studies: newborn screening for hypothyroidism; then annual T4, TSH throughout childhood and adulthood
- Vision screening at age 4 years

These guidelines are published and maintained by the AAP.

Future Risk of Sibling with Down Syndrome

If the child has 3 complete copies of chromosome 21 and the mother is < 35 years of age, her risk of having another child with trisomy 21 is 1%. If the mother is > 35 years of age, the risk is similar to the age-specific risk.

If the child with trisomy 21 has Down syndrome due to an unbalanced translocation, the future risk depends on the parents' cytogenetic analysis. The other chromosomes involved determine risk of recurrence. For example, if a

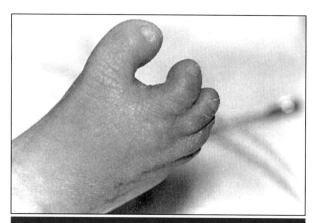

Figure 9-7: Trisomy 21, Brachydactyly & Broad Space

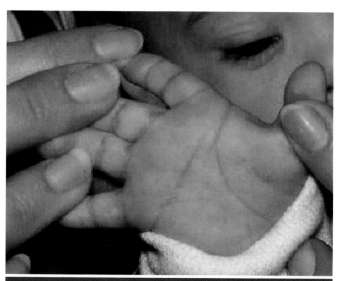

Figure 9-8: Trisomy 21, Single Palmar Crease

notes

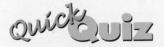

Quick Quiz

1) What are the common congenital heart defects found in a child with trisomy 21?

2) What GI defects are associated with trisomy 21?

3) What glandular disorder should you annually screen for in children/adults with trisomy 21?

4) What should be done at age 3 to assess the spine in children with trisomy 21?

5) A 30-year-old mother has a child with trisomy 21 with 3 complete copies of chromosome 21. What is her risk of having another child with trisomy 21?

6) Is trisomy 18 more common in boys or girls?

7) What are the classic features of a child with trisomy 18?

8) What are the classic features of a child with trisomy 13?

parent has a 21:21 translocation, the risk of having an offspring with Down syndrome would be 100%. However, in general, if the father has a balanced translocation, the recurrence risk is 1–2%; if the mother has a balanced translocation, the recurrence risk is 10–15%.

TRISOMY 18 (EDWARDS SYNDROME)

Trisomy 18 is the second most common autosomal trisomy and occurs in about 1/6,000 live births, with a much higher incidence of stillbirths. The ratio of girls to boys born with Edwards syndrome is 4:1. The risk of having an offspring with trisomy 18 becomes more prevalent as maternal age increases. 95% of cases are due to 3 copies of chromosome 18, with the other 5% due to mosaicism or partial trisomy of the long arm of 18. The risk of recurrence for future pregnancies is less than 1% (less than for full trisomy 21 cases) for mothers < 35 years of age; it is age-specific for older mothers.

Characteristic findings of trisomy 18:
- Intrauterine growth restriction
- Mental retardation
- High forehead
- Microcephaly
- Small face and mouth
- Short sternum
- Rocker bottom feet (see Figure 9-9)
- Clubfoot/clenched fist (see Figure 9-9)
- Overlapping fingers
- Hypoplastic nails
- Structural heart defects (90%): most often a VSD with multiple dysplastic valves

50% of affected children die in the 1st week of life, with another 40% dying by 1 year of age. Most die because of central apnea. Children with trisomy 18 do not learn to walk or develop language skills. Those who survive past 1 year of age typically function on a 6–12-month-old level, although some may develop skills up to the level of a 2-year-old.

TRISOMY 13 (PATAU SYNDROME)

Trisomy 13 is the third most common autosomal trisomy in humans and occurs in about 1/20,000–1/25,000 live births. 80% of children with trisomy 13 have 3 complete copies, and the remaining have 3 copies of the long arm of 13 due to an unbalanced translocation. Very few trisomy 13 children are mosaic. Recurrence risk for trisomy 13 is presumed to be very low and, similar to trisomy 18, < 1% for a mother < 35 years of age. Again, it is age-specific for older mothers.

Common clinical findings in trisomy 13 include (Think midline defects!):
- Orofacial cleft (often midline cleft lip—see Figure 9-10)
- Microphthalmia
- Postaxial polydactyly of the limbs (see Figure 9-11)
- Holoprosencephaly (cyclopia to premaxillary agenesis)
- Heart malformations (80%)
- Hypoplastic or absent ribs
- Genital anomalies
- Abdominal-wall defects
- Cutis aplasia

Median survival for children with trisomy 13 is 2.5 days. Approximately 80% of babies die within the first month, and only 5% survive the first 6 months. Survivors have severe mental retardation, seizures, and failure to thrive.

MOSAIC TRISOMY 8

Trisomy 8 is (relatively) the rarest of the trisomies. Of those who are born live, it is usually seen as mosaic trisomy 8. Diagnosis is usually made only by performing chromosome

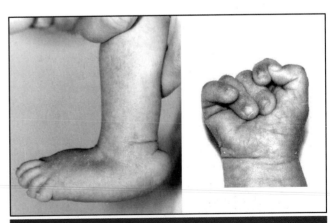

Figure 9-9: Trisomy 18 (Edwards Syndrome)

notes

analysis on skin fibroblasts (to detect chromosomal mosaicism). These children have a long face, high forehead, a thick, everted lower lip, deep palmar and sole creases (very characteristic finding), and low-set ears. Bone, joint, and renal malformations are common. These children are at increased risk of AML at older ages.

DELETION SYNDROMES
OVERVIEW

Deletions occur when a piece of chromosome is missing. It can occur as a simple "stand alone" deletion or as a deletion with duplication of another chromosome segment. Most deletion syndromes present as mental retardation with associated phenotypic anomalies. If the deletion comes from the short arm, it is denoted as "p-"; from the long arm, it is denoted as "q-".

4p- (WOLF-HIRSCHHORN SYNDROME)

4p-deletion occurs in about 1/50,000 births and is most common in girls. Most (~ 87%) cases are *de novo*, while 13% are due to one of the parents having a balanced chromosome translocation.

Features:
* "Greek helmet" facies (ocular hypertelorism, prominent glabella, and frontal bossing)
* Growth deficiency
* Microcephaly
* "Beaked" nose
* Hypertension
* Short philtrum
* Hypotonia
* Congenital cardiac anomalies (50%)
* Seizures (90%)

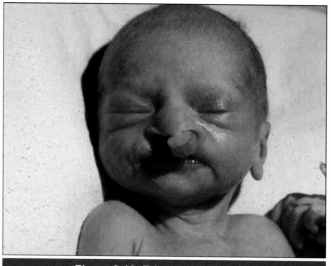

Figure 9-10: Trisomy 13, Cleft Lip

Most of these children have profound developmental delay, but some can walk unsupported and even speak a few phrases.

5p- (CRI-DU-CHAT SYNDROME)

5p-, or cri-du-chat syndrome, is due to a deletion of the short arm of chromosome 5. This is always on the Board exam, so be sure to know it! It is well known because of the association with the distinctive "cat's cry," which is due to an anatomic change in the larynx.

Characteristics of this syndrome:
* "Moon face" with telecanthus (widely spaced eyes) in infancy and early childhood
* Down-slanting palpebral fissures
* Hypotonia
* Short stature
* Microcephaly
* High-arched palate
* Wide and flat nasal bridge
* Mental retardation

Cardiac manifestations occur in about 33% of affected children.

18q- (De GROUCHY SYNDROME)

18q-, or De Grouchy syndrome, is due to deletion of the long arm of chromosome 18. The main characteristics are microcephaly and developmental delay.

Other characteristics:
* Atretic or narrowed ear canals (classic)
* "Frog-like" position with legs flexed, externally rotated, and in hyperabduction
* Depressed midface
* Protruding mandible
* Deep-set eyes
* Everted lower lip (carp-like mouth)
* Mental retardation

OTHER DELETIONS

There are numerous other deletions, but those listed above are the most commonly tested on the Boards. Others listed in major pediatric textbooks include:

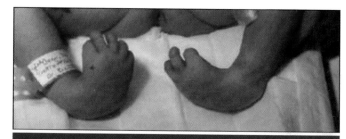

Figure 9-11: Trisomy 13; Postaxial Polydactyly

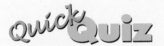

- 9p-: trigonocephaly (triangle head), discrete exophthalmos, arched eyebrows, short neck with pterygium colli (a bilateral web or tight band of skin of the neck, extending from the acromion to the mastoid), long fingers and toes, and cardiac abnormalities.
- 13q-: low birthweight, FTT, severe mental retardation; ocular manifestations are common; hypoplastic hands and absent thumbs with syndactyly.
- 18p-: 80% of those affected will have only mild retardation and minor anomalies; 20% will have severe ocular and brain abnormalities (including holoprosencephaly), cleft lip/palate, and mental retardation. IgA deficiency is found in a majority of these patients.
- 21q-: large, low-set ears, micrognathia, hypertonia, downward-slanting palpebral fissures; skeletal abnormalities.

MICRODELETION OR CONTIGUOUS GENE SYNDROMES

OVERVIEW

Microdeletions are small chromosome deletions that are detectable only in high-quality (pro-) metaphase preparations or with fluorescent *in situ* hybridization (FISH) directed at specific regions known to be missing in various disorders. These deletions often involve several genes ("contiguous gene deletion syndromes"), so that you may also identify affected individuals with more "typical" phenotypes associated with single gene mutations, such as Duchenne muscular dystrophy. FISH identifies microdeletions (see Williams syndrome).

A recent addition to the testing for microdeletions and microduplications is known as chromosomal microarray analysis (CMA), or array comparative genomic hybridization, which provides whole genome coverage. Oligonucleotide microarray technology has a 6,000-band karyotype equivalent and the ability to identify deletions or duplications as small as 500 kb anywhere in the genome. It targets all telomere, centromere, and known microdeletion/microduplication syndromes. Compared to standard G-banded karyotype (500–650 bands), it can detect deletions and duplications of ~ 5 Mb (CMA therefore provides ~ 10x better resolution). All imbalances are confirmed by a second methodology (usually FISH analysis).

There are multiple newly identified, but less well-described, microdeletion/microduplication syndromes.

15q11–13 (ANGELMAN AND PRADER-WILLI SYNDROMES)

Maternal vs. Paternal

Although we discussed these syndromes earlier under the genomic imprinting topic, 15q11–13 microdeletion deserves special attention because it is such a common topic on the Board exam. Remember: This deletion's phenotypic appearance depends solely on whether it is maternally (Angelman) or paternally (Prader-Willi) derived.

Maternally Derived 15q11–13 (Angelman Syndrome)

Classic findings:
- Jerky ataxic movements (the "happy puppet," but do not use this nomenclature except to remember for the Board exam!)
- Characteristic gait
- Hypotonia
- Fair hair
- Midface hypoplasia
- Prognathism (large chin, mandible)
- Seizures
- Inappropriate bouts of laughter
- Severe mental retardation
- Absent or severely delayed speech

Paternally Derived 15q11–13 (Prader-Willi Syndrome)

Classic findings:
- Severe hypotonia at birth
- Obesity (after failure to thrive initially)
- Short stature
- Small hands and feet
- Hypogonadism
- Usually mild mental retardation

(See Figure 9-12.)

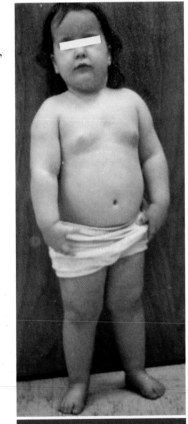

Figure 9-12: Prader-Willi Synd.

7q11.23- (WILLIAMS SYNDROME)

Williams syndrome, due to microdeletion on the long arm of chromosome 7, has the following characteristic features and facies (see Figure 9-13):
• Periorbital fullness with prominent, down-turned lower lip
• Friendly "cocktail party" personality
• Stellate pattern of the iris
• Strabismus
• Supravalvular aortic stenosis
• Mental retardation
• Hypercalcemia

In 95% or more of the cases studied, individuals having Williams syndrome are missing the elastin gene from one of their two copies of chromosome number 7. The FISH technique will detect the absence of an elastin gene from a chromosome. FISH is an acronym for the technical expression fluorescence *in situ* hybridization. For Williams syndrome, you take a blood sample from the child and then treat the sample with 2 specifically colored markers that give off a "fluorescent" light when exposed to ultraviolet light. One of the markers attaches to each of the two copies of chromosome 7 in a cell. When both copies of chromosome 7 possess the elastin gene, you can see an additional fluorescence of another color attached at another location to each of the two copies of chromosome 7. But, as is the case in over 95% of those with Williams syndrome, only one copy of chromosome 7, not two, will show the fluorescent spot for the elastin gene.

11p13- (WAGR SYNDROME)

11p13- deletion results in WAGR syndrome: Wilms tumor, Aniridia, Genitourinary malformations, and mental Retardation. It occurs due to the absence of 2 possible genes, *PAX6* and *Wilms tumor 1 (WT1)*.

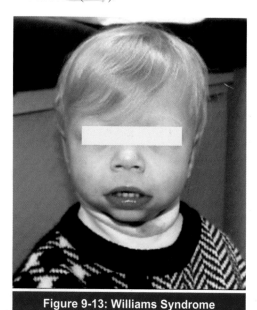

Figure 9-13: Williams Syndrome

Characteristics of WAGR syndrome:
• Wilms tumor (Wilms tumor occurs in up to 50% of cases, most often by 3 years of age)
• Aniridia
• Male genital hypoplasia (hypospadias, cryptorchidism, small penis, and/or hypoplastic scrotum)
• Mental retardation (the majority of patients have some degree of mental retardation, although the range is very wide (from IQ < 35 to normal functioning)
• Gonadoblastoma
• Long face
• Upward-slanting palpebral fissures
• Ptosis
• Beaked nose
• Poorly formed ears

20p12- (ALAGILLE SYNDROME)

20p12- deletion, or Alagille syndrome, has AD inheritance and is caused by mutation in the *Jagged-1 (JAG1)* gene.

Characteristics include:
• Bile duct paucity with cholestasis
• Pulmonary valve stenosis and peripheral artery stenoses
• Ocular defects (posterior embryotoxon—a developmental abnormality marked by a prominent white ring of Schwalbe and iris strands that partially obscure the chamber angle)
• Skeletal defects: butterfly vertebrae
• Triangular facies with pointed chin
• Long nose with broad mid-nose

Hepatic involvement typically presents in the first 3 months of life as cholestasis, jaundice, and pruritus, with a paucity of bile ducts observed histologically; some patients develop liver failure. The most common cardiac manifestations are peripheral and branch pulmonic stenosis (67% of patients) and tetralogy of Fallot (7–16% of patients). Posterior embryotoxon (prominent Schwalbe ring) of the eye and butterfly vertebrae do not generally cause symptoms.

22q11.2- (VELOCARDIOFACIAL/DiGEORGE SYNDROME)

The 22q11.2- deletion syndrome includes phenotypes referred to as DiGeorge syndrome, Shprintzen syndrome, velocardiofacial (VCF) syndrome, or CATCH 22 (Cleft palate, Absent Thymus, Congenital Heart disease—this mnemonic/term is no longer used, because it is derogatory, but for Board purposes it may help you remember). It is probably best designated as "22q11.2 deletion syndrome."

Characteristics include:
• Cleft palate, velopharyngeal incompetence (VPI)
• Thymus agenesis or hypoplasia (immune deficiencies)
• Parathyroid gland hypoplasia/agenesis (hypocalcemia)

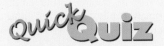

- Hypoplasia of the auricle and external auditory canal
- Cardiac abnormalities in decreasing order of frequency: tetralogy of Fallot > interrupted aortic arch > VSD > truncus arteriosus
- Short stature
- Behavioral problems

This is a developmental defect of derivatives of the 3rd and 4th pharyngeal pouches, associated with agenesis or hypoplasia of the thymus and parathyroid gland, conotruncal heart defects, and branchial arch defects (small chin, cleft palate, abnormal ears). A majority of patients with 22q11.2 deletion have hypotonia in infancy and learning disabilities, with nonverbal learning disability in ~ 66% of patients and ~ 20–30% having mental retardation. Presentation varies widely even within families, ranging from isolated psychiatric disorders or learning problems to severe congenital heart defects.

SEX CHROMOSOME ABNORMALITIES

INCIDENCE

About 1/500 neonates has an abnormality of either the X or the Y chromosome. 47,XXY (Klinefelter syndrome), 47,XYY, and 47,XXX make up 80% of this group. Turner syndrome is much less common, occurring in only about 1/2,500 to 1/5,000 neonate females.

47,XXY (KLINEFELTER SYNDROME)

47,XXY (Klinefelter syndrome) presents with a male phenotype and an extra X chromosome. (See Figure 9-14.)

Most cases are not associated with advanced maternal age. Meiotic nondisjunction is a common cause, with the extra X chromosome mostly of maternal origin. Usually, these patients are quite tall with gynecomastia, and secondary sex development is delayed. They almost always have azoospermia, small testes, and are infertile. Klinefelter syndrome is discussed in more detail in the Endocrinology section.

OTHER EXTRA X CHROMOSOME SYNDROMES

There are many other syndromes in which 1 or more extra X chromosomes occur: 47,XXX; 48,XXXX; 49,XXXXX; 48,XXXY; and 49,XXXXY. Frequently, they are mosaic with a "normal" 46,XX and an abnormal cell line (for example, 46,XX/47,XXX). As the number of X chromosomes increases, the degree of phenotypic abnormality increases; specifically, the neurological problems are worse.

47,XYY MALE

47,XYY occurs in about 1/1,000 live births. XYY males are generally taller than average. Otherwise, this is no longer considered a true syndrome. Earlier studies suggesting increased behavior problems have now been documented to be "flawed;" and these males are not different from the general population.

45,X (TURNER SYNDROME)

Turner syndrome is discussed in detail in the Endocrinology section. (See Figure 9-15 and Figure 9-16.)

These girls are phenotypically female and have short stature and ovarian failure/gonadal dysgenesis with subsequent lack of secondary sexual development. About 5–10% have some Y chromosome material in all or some cells, which puts them at risk for gonadoblastoma. Other chromosome abnormalities found in patients with Turner syndrome include:
- Deletion Xp, deletion Xq, ring X (r(X))
- Mosaics: 45,X/46,XX; 45,X/46,X,i(Xq)
- 46,X,i(Xq)

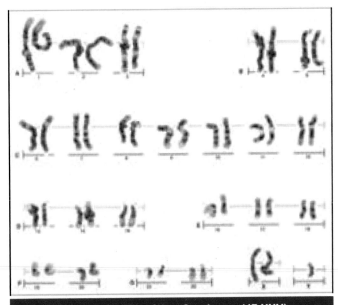

Figure 9-14: Klinefelter Syndrome (47,XXY)

notes

Also remember that about 50% of these girls have cardiovascular anomalies, including bicuspid aortic valves, and 15–20% have coarctation of the aorta. Other findings at birth include broad, webbed neck (from fetal cystic hygroma), posteriorly rotated ears, lymphedema of the hands and feet, and cubitus valgus. Other common associated disorders in childhood or adulthood are: Hashimoto thyroiditis, alopecia, carbohydrate intolerance, vitiligo, and gastrointestinal disorders. 99% of fetuses with Turner syndrome spontaneously abort.

CHROMOSOMAL INSTABILITY SYNDROMES

Chromosomal instability syndromes refer to a group of disorders that are largely AR and have an increased frequency of chromosomal breaks. These include ataxia-telangiectasia, Bloom syndrome, Fanconi syndrome, and xeroderma pigmentosum. These are discussed in other sections.

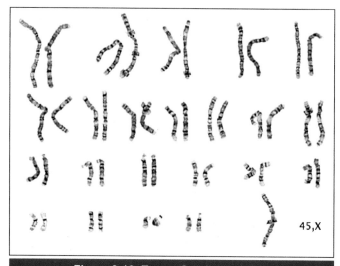

Figure 9-15: Turner Syndrome (45,X)

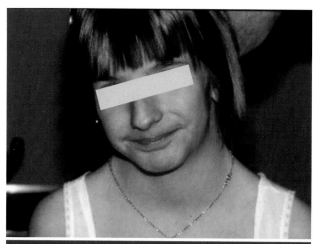

45,X

Figure 9-16: Turner Syndrome (45,X)

At the end of this section is a set of tables listing common congenital anomaly syndromes (and/or other syndromes sometimes tested on the Board exam); see Table 9-3 through Table 9-11.

ANOMALIES OF THE HEAD
CLEFT LIP / PALATE DISORDERS

Cleft lip and/or cleft palate is one of the most common craniofacial malformations you will see in your practice. The incidence varies from 1/250 to 1/3,000, depending on the culture and race being reviewed. Native Americans have the highest rates, and African-Americans have the lowest rates.

Most cases of cleft lip/palate are sporadic, but there can be recurrence in families, and hereditary factors have been documented. If the first-born child has a cleft lip/palate, the risk of the next sibling having it is 3–4%. If either parent had one as a child, the risk goes up further. There are nearly 300 syndromes associated with cleft lip/palate—make sure you know all 300 very well. (Just kidding!)

Airway management and feeding difficulties are the usual problems at birth. These children are at risk for recurrent otitis media and persistent middle-ear effusions.

Generally, surgically repair the lip within the first 5 months of life, and repair a cleft palate at 6–12 months of age.

The following 2 sequences are important to know for the Boards! "Sequence" refers to a pattern of anomalies that results from a single identifiable event in development.

Pierre-Robin Sequence

Pierre-Robin sequence presents with a primary embryologic defect of mandibular hypoplasia, which leads to displacement of the tongue, interrupted closure of the lateral palatine ridges, and cleft palate. Patients have glossoptosis (downward displacement of the tongue), micrognathia, respiratory distress, and feeding problems.

Amniotic Band Sequence

Amniotic band sequence can present with disruptive clefts of the face and palate resulting from amniotic bands becoming adherent to any part of the fetal body. Other defects can include constriction rings of the limbs and/or digits and amputations.

HEMIFACIAL MICROSOMIA

Findings

The second most common craniofacial malformation is the association of external ear anomalies (microtia—smallness of the auricle of the ear with a blind or absent external auditory meatus; anotia—congenital absence of one or both auricles of the ears; canal atresia; and/or preauricular tags) with maxillary and/or mandibular hypoplasia.

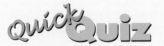
The malformations can occur as isolated events or be part of a malformation "syndrome." Cervical vertebral anomalies occur in nearly 33% with hemifacial microsomia, and cardiac anomalies occur frequently as well. Also be aware that renal anomalies occur in about 15% of those with these ear malformations, so a renal ultrasound may be a good answer on the Board exam when they ask what further studies are warranted.

Goldenhar syndrome (see below) and hemifacial microsomia are considered to be the same disorder; but use the term Goldenhar syndrome only if epibulbar dermoids are present.

Goldenhar Syndrome

A child with Goldenhar syndrome has all of the findings of hemifacial microsomia mentioned above. The patient presents with hemifacial microsomia, epibulbar lipodermoids (lateral-inferior, fibrous-fatty masses on the globe), vertebral defects, cardiac anomalies (VSD or outflow tract malformations), and renal anomalies. Preauricular and facial tags are common. You also will see conductive hearing loss. This syndrome most commonly occurs as a "sporadic" finding, but some propose AD inheritance in some families. The cause is unknown, but some cases are reported to be due to vascular interruption during embryonic development.

OTHER FACIAL ANOMALY SYNDROMES

Branchio-Oto-Renal (BOR) Syndrome

BOR syndrome presents with branchial cleft fistulas or cysts, preauricular pits, cochlear and stapes malformation, mixed sensory and conductive hearing loss, and renal dysplasia/aplasia. Occasionally, patients will have pulmonary hypoplasia. It is inherited as an AD disorder.

Treacher-Collins Syndrome
(Mandibulofacial Dysostosis Type 1)

Treacher-Collins syndrome is another AD disorder and presents with mandibular and maxillary hypoplasia, zygomatic arch clefts, and various forms of ear malformations (microtia, anotia, atresia). Other characteristic findings include down-sloping palpebral fissures and colobomata of the lower eyelids. Conductive hearing loss is also common.

CRANIOSYNOSTOSIS

Craniosynostosis occurs sporadically in 1/2,000 live births; 1/25,000 cases are hereditary. Craniosynostosis is the early, pathologic fusion of calvarial sutures. The most common, single-suture fusion is sagittal synostosis. The others, in descending order, are coronal > metopic > lambdoid. Isolated lambdoid is very rare, occurring in only 2–3% of cases. Sagittal synostosis is more common in males by a ratio of 5:1.

What shapes form from the different early fusions?
- Sagittal sutures: result in excessive anterior/posterior growth with a resulting long, narrow head shape with frontal and occipital prominence, known as scaphocephaly.
- Coronal and sphenofrontal sutures: result in unilateral flattening of the forehead, elevation of the ipsilateral orbit and eyebrow, and a prominent ear on the affected side, known as frontal plagiocephaly. More common in girls.
- Metopic sutures: result in keel-shaped forehead and hypotelorism; known as trigonocephaly.
- Coronal, sphenofrontal, and frontoethmoidal sutures: cause a cone-shaped head; known as turricephaly.

There is more on craniosynostosis in The Fetus & Newborn section.

Syndromic hereditary forms exist, including Apert and Crouzon syndromes, which are discussed briefly in Table 9-3 at the end of this section. You can distinguish many of these from each other by particular hand malformations. You must surgically intervene to correct the risk of intracranial hypertension, as well as repair facial asymmetry and make the shape of the head more normal.

PLAGIOCEPHALY
(Positional Flattening of the Skull)

Positional flattening of the skull (plagiocephaly) occurs postnatally and is caused by the infant's positional preference of sleeping/resting. It is frequently associated with torticollis and can cause flattening of the occipitoparietal area. It may be severe enough to cause ipsilateral frontal prominence or anterior displacement of the ipsilateral ear.

It can look like lambdoid synostosis, but you can differentiate it by physical examination and, if necessary, skull CT, where lambdoid synostosis shows sclerosis of the lambdoid suture. On the Board exam, be on the lookout for this: Lambdoid synostosis is rare, while positional plagiocephaly is common.

Things to look for in positional plagiocephaly: anterior displacement of the ipsilateral ear (posterior/inferior for lambdoid); ipsilateral frontal prominence (absent in lambdoid); absent contralateral occipitoparietal prominence (present in lambdoid); no lambdoid ridge or sub-mastoid prominence (present in lambdoid); and positional plagiocephaly stops progressing after 7 months, since children generally can roll over and move their head more (lambdoid continues to progress after 7 months). Positional plagiocephaly has become more common since we've started recommending "back to sleep," and improves with "tummy time."

Usually, you do not need to treat positional plagiocephaly. Special "helmets" for sleeping are available in severe cases.

SKELETAL DYSPLASIAS
ACHONDROPLASIA

Achondroplasia, the most common skeletal dysplasia, occurs in 1/20,000 live births and consists of:

• disproportionately short stature with rhizomelic shortening (short lengths of the most proximal segment of the upper arms and legs compared to the distal segments),
• trident hands,
• macrocephaly, and
• characteristic craniofacial findings, including a flat nasal bridge, prominent forehead, and midfacial hypoplasia. (See Figure 9-17.)

It is an AD disorder with most having a *de novo* mutation of *FGFR3* (fibroblast growth factor receptor 3) on chromosome 4p16.3. This gain-of-function mutation results in decreased endochondral ossification, decreased chondrocyte proliferation, and cartilage matrix production, which results in glycine residue replaced by an arginine.

The hands have a "trident" appearance: the hands are short and the fingers are quite broad, with digits 3 and 4 splayed more distally than proximally. These children are on the growth curve at birth, but by age 2–3 months their length has fallen to < 5th percentile. Note that children with achondroplasia usually do not have other malformations.

Confirm diagnosis with characteristic x-ray findings: squared-off iliac wings, flat and irregular acetabulum roofs, thick femoral necks, and "ice-cream-scoop-shaped" femoral heads, as well as the rhizomelic shortening mentioned above.

These children are at increased risk for serous otitis media, motor milestone delay, bowing of the legs, and orthodontic problems. Most males have final heights of 118–145 cm and females of 112–136 cm.

Foramen magnum stenosis and/or craniocervical junction abnormalities can occur in infancy and cause compression of the upper cord—resulting in apnea, quadriparesis, growth delay, and hydrocephalus. The AAP recommends measuring the size and shape of the fontanelle and monthly monitor-

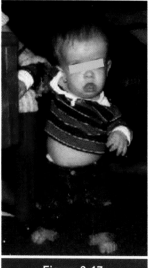

Figure 9-17: Achondroplasia

ing of the occipitofrontal circumference.

This disorder is usually the result of a new mutation, and the mutation rate increases with advancing paternal age.

THANATOPHORIC DYSPLASIAS

Thanatophoric dysplasias Types 1 and 2 also involve mutations of *FGFR3*, but most cases are lethal. Both are AD and almost always due to *de novo* mutations. Death is due either to compression of the cervicomedullary region of the foramen magnum or to pulmonary hypoplasia.

Those affected have macrocephaly with very short limbs. X-ray is diagnostic, showing platyspondyly (flatness of the bodies of the vertebrae), flared metaphyses of the long bones, and short iliac bones. Type 1 has bowed femurs, while Type 2 exhibits straight femurs. Also, the Type 2 infants have a "cloverleaf" skull.

CARTILAGE ANOMALIES
OSTEOGENESIS IMPERFECTA

All Types

Osteogenesis imperfecta refers to a disorder characterized by osseous fragility, short stature, and skeletal findings that vary based on the type. There are 4 recognized forms of osteogenesis imperfecta, all of which are caused by autosomal dominant genetic defects affecting collagen. None of these forms causes retinal hemorrhage or subdural hematomas, which distinguishes osteogenesis imperfecta from abuse.

Osteogenesis Imperfecta Type I

Osteogenesis imperfecta Type I is an AD disease that is also known as "brittle bone disease." It is the mildest and most common type of osteogenesis imperfecta. Common characteristics include:

• Blue sclerae
• Delayed fontanelle closure
• Hyperextensible joints
• Hearing loss
• Stature (usually normal or near normal)
• Multiple fractures (most occur before puberty)

Fractures rarely occur at birth but are frequent in childhood, especially with even minor trauma. By adolescence, the fracture frequency diminishes. X-rays show mild osteopenia of the long bones and wormian bones (bones without sutures). Other associated manifestations of scoliosis and hearing loss appear in the 20s and 30s. There is a decrease in synthesis of Type 1 collagen.

Osteogenesis Imperfecta Type II

Osteogenesis imperfecta Type II, the most severe form, results in death during the newborn period due to respiratory insufficiency. These children have numerous fractures and severe bone deformity. The skull is very soft, and the limbs are short and bowed. X-ray shows long bones with a "crumpled

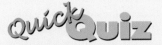

appearance," and the ribs are beaded due to callus formation. Almost all cases are due to *de novo* AD mutation of the *COL1A1* gene, which disrupts collagen formation.

Osteogenesis Imperfecta Type III

Osteogenesis imperfecta Type III presents in the newborn with numerous fractures. We used to call this the progressively deforming type. Short stature is severe, and many cannot ambulate because they can't bear their own weight. Blue sclerae occur at birth but lighten with age—unlike those in Type I, which stay dark blue. Most cases are due to a point mutation of the *COL1A1* gene, similar to Type II. Neurologic complications are most common with Type III, including hydrocephalus and basilar skull invagination.

Osteogenesis Imperfecta Type IV

Osteogenesis imperfecta Type IV is a milder form, like Type I. The sclerae are usually white or near-white. Fontanelle closure is delayed, and fractures are present at birth. These individuals have shorter-than-average stature. Tibial bowing is the hallmark of Type IV. Children with this type and Type I have dentinogenesis imperfecta. Most patients with Type IV have a point mutation of the *COL1A2* gene.

CONNECTIVE TISSUE DYSPLASIAS
MARFAN SYNDROME

Marfan syndrome is an AD disorder that affects 1/5,000 individuals. Boys and girls are affected equally. The affected organ systems include the eyes, circulatory system, skeleton, skin, lungs, and dura. Most deaths occur due to cardiac complications, namely aortic root dilation and rupture.

The red-highlighted areas in Table 9-1 are frequently clues to a patient on the Board exam with Marfan syndrome. Look for the child with "high-arched palate, dislocated lens, pectus carinatum or excavatum, and mitral valve prolapse." (See Figure 9-18 and Figure 9-19.)

Diagnosis is still made by clinical findings, even though fibrillin gene testing is available. Diagnosis in a patient without an affected 1st degree relative requires major manifestations in at least 2 different organ systems and minor criteria in a 3rd. If there is a documented 1st degree relative, only 1 major and 1 minor manifestation in a 2nd organ system are required. Also, the presence of a mutation in the gene that encodes fibrillin-1, *FBN1*, is a major criterion. Always rule out homocystinuria, which has many features similar to Marfan syndrome, by checking for the absence of homocystine in the urine (without pyridoxine supplementation).

Since cardiovascular complications are the most serious, annual or semi-annual echocardiograms are the norm. Additionally, beta-blockade will slow aortic dilation, especially in children. These children should avoid weightlifting and strenuous exercise, but aerobic, noncompetitive exercise is important.

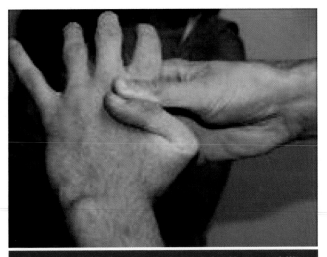

Figure 9-18: Marfan Syndrome—Joint Hypermobility

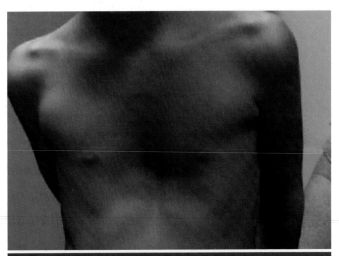

Figure 9-19: Marfan Syndrome—Pectus Excavatum

notes

Some have advocated inducing puberty early with exogenous hormones to limit the degree of curvature and deformity, caused by scoliosis or kyphoscoliosis, and to reduce final adult height. Most especially recommend this for girls whose final projected adult height is greater than 6 feet. Pregnancy increases the risk of accelerated aortic dilatation in women with Marfan syndrome.

EHLERS-DANLOS SYNDROMES

Ehlers-Danlos syndromes are a group of autosomal dominant connective tissue disorders that generally include hyperextensible skin, hypermobile joints, easy bruising, and dystrophic scarring. There are 6 major variants, with varying characteristics. For the Boards, you really need to know only the "classic" type, which represents the majority of cases.

The skin findings are classic (Know!), and some describe the skin's texture as "wet chamois" or a "fine sponge." "Extra" skin is common over the hands, feet, and stomach. The skin is very stretchy and returns to its normal configuration on release, much like a rubber band. The skin is unusually fragile and can split with the slightest trauma, especially at the shins, knees, elbows, and chin. There generally is not a lot of bleeding, but the skin will have a gaping "fish-mouth" appearance at the tear. Scarring is abnormal, and scars that appear are usually thin and shiny. Increased bruising is common, especially in children, as is bleeding from the gums after tooth-brushing. All coagulation tests (including PT, PTT, bleeding time) are normal, except for capillary fragility

Table 9-1: Major and Minor Findings of Marfan Syndrome	
Major Manifestations	
Skeletal	- Pectus carinatum (flattening of the chest on either side with forward projection of the sternum resembling the keel of a boat; "pigeon breast") - Pectus excavatum (a hollow at the lower part of the chest caused by a backward displacement of the xiphoid cartilage; "funnel chest") severe enough to require surgery - Reduced upper and lower segment ratio or arm-span-to-height ratio - Wrist sign (overlapping of the thumb and 5th finger when encircling the wrist) - Thumb sign (extension of the thumb past the ulnar border of the hand when opposed to the palm) - Pes planus (a condition in which the longitudinal arch is broken down, with the entire sole touching the ground; "flat foot") - Scoliosis > 20% - Reduced extension of the elbows (< 170%) - Protrusio acetabuli (characterized by an inward bulging of the acetabulum into the pelvic cavity)
Ocular	- Ectopia lentis (displacement of the lens of the eye)
Cardiovascular	- Dilation of the ascending aorta - Dissection of the ascending aorta
Dura	- Lumbosacral dural ectasia (dilation)
Minor Manifestations	
Skeletal	- Moderate pectus excavatum - Joint hypermobility - High-arched palate
Ocular	- Abnormally flat cornea - Hypoplastic iris or ciliary muscle
Cardiovascular	- Mitral valve prolapse - Dilation of the main pulmonary artery
Pulmonary	- Spontaneous pneumothorax - Apical blebs
Skin	- Striae atrophicae (bands of thin wrinkled skin, initially red but becoming purple and white, which occur commonly on the abdomen, buttocks, and thighs; these result from atrophy of the dermis and overextension of the skin) - Recurrent or incisional hernias

notes

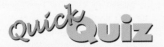

1) Describe the classic findings in Ehlers-Danlos syndrome.

2) What are the classic skin findings in neurofibromatosis Type 1?

3) By what inheritance pattern do a majority of neurofibromatosis cases appear in a population?

4) Describe how neurofibromatosis Type 2 differs from neurofibromatosis Type 1.

testing. Wrinkled palms and soles are common, as are pseudotumors at the heels, elbows, and knees from abnormal scarring.

Joint hypermobility is common but may not occur in certain types. Both large and small joints can be involved. Dislocations are common and can be present at birth. Knees and elbows can be extended past 180°, and the fingers can be extended past 90°. The joint mobility decreases with increasing age.

Mitral valve prolapse and proximal aortic dilatation occur; screen for these with echocardiogram, CT, or MRI.

Aim treatment at prevention with the use of shin guards, high-topped boots, and kneepads. Forbid physical contact sports.

NEUROCUTANEOUS DISEASES
NEUROFIBROMATOSIS TYPE 1

Neurofibromatosis Type 1 (formerly known as von Recklinghausen disease) is the most common neurocutaneous disease and affects about 1/2,000. Classically, café-au-lait spots and benign cutaneous neurofibromas characterize Type 1 disease.

Table 9-2: Clinical Criteria for Neurofibromatosis Type 1

≥ 6 café-au-lait spots of > 0.5 cm in greatest diameter in prepubertal children, and > 1.5 cm in post-pubertal

≥ 2 neurofibromas of any type or 1 plexiform neurofibroma

Freckling in the axillary or inguinal areas

Optic glioma

≥ 2 Lisch nodules (iris hamartomas)

Sphenoid dysplasia or thinning of the long bone cortex with or without pseudarthrosis

1st degree relative (parent, sibling, child) with neurofibromatosis Type 1

Most children have diagnostic findings by age 10. Specific diagnosis requires 2 of 7 criteria. See Table 9-2 for a list of the clinical criteria.

The café-au-lait spots (see Figure 9-20) usually appear in the first 2 years of life, but don't forget that these also may appear with other syndromes, such as McCune-Albright syndrome. The axillary freckles appear by adolescence in 75% (see Figure 9-21). You also will see the Lisch nodules (iris hamartomas) in about 75% of prepubescent children.

What are neurofibromas? They are benign, peripheral nerve sheath tumors that are a collection of Schwann-like cells, fibroblasts, and extracellular matrices. The cutaneous neurofibromas appear at puberty, while the plexiform neurofibromas are present before then and are usually congenital.

The bony changes occur in early childhood years and include sphenoid wing dysplasia, long-bone bowing, and dysplastic scoliosis.

About 50% of affected children have learning disorders or speech impediments. Other features to look for include short stature, macrocephaly, hypertension, constipation, and headaches.

Nearly 60% of cases are sporadic or *de novo* AD mutations, but once established, it is AD in inheritance. The phenotypic expression is quite variable from one affected individual to another, even among family members. The gene, *neurofibromin*, maps to chromosome 17.

NEUROFIBROMATOSIS TYPE 2

Neurofibromatosis Type 2 is also an AD disorder characterized by the presence of bilateral vestibular schwannomas (acoustic neuromas). Type 1 and Type 2 are very distinct and different disorders, with no commonality with regard to genetic factors. Type 2 is much less common than Type 1 and has an incidence of about 1/40,000–1/50,000. The mean age for clinical presentation is 30 years, but children are frequently diagnosed with the disorder. The vestibular

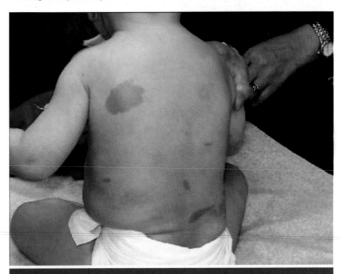

Figure 9-20: Neurofibromatosis Type 1, Café-au-Lait Spots

notes

schwannomas cause hearing loss, tinnitus, imbalance, and facial weakness. Other CNS tumors occur in about 50% of cases and include intracranial meningiomas, spinal schwannomas, cranial nerve schwannomas (5th cranial nerve most commonly), and ependymomas. Lens opacities or cataracts occur as one of the first signs and can be used for screening in children. Diagnostic criteria: the presence of either bilateral acoustic neuromas alone or a 1st degree relative with neurofibromatosis Type 2 and either unilateral acoustic neuroma, two of the previous CNS tumors, or lenticular opacity. Neurofibromatosis Type 2 has been mapped to chromosome 22. For relatives at risk, do MRI screening to detect vestibular schwannomas small enough to be surgically removed, and thus preserve hearing.

TUBEROUS SCLEROSIS

Tuberous sclerosis is an AD disorder that may affect 1/6,000 people. There are many features of tuberous sclerosis, but the classic findings are:

- Ash leaf hypopigmented macules (most common presentation in ~ 90% of cases; see Figure 9-22)
- Shagreen patches (an oval-shaped nevoid plaque, skin-colored or occasionally pigmented, smooth or crinkled, appearing on the trunk or lower back)
- Facial angiomas
- Forehead plaques
- Ungual (nail) and gingival fibromas
- Polycystic kidney disease associated with *TSC2* (on chromosome 16)

Tuberous sclerosis has wide variability, both between and within families, much like the variability you see with neurofibromatosis Type 1. Some of the features you may find in early childhood disappear by adulthood, making diagnosis more difficult. For example, nearly 50% of infants have

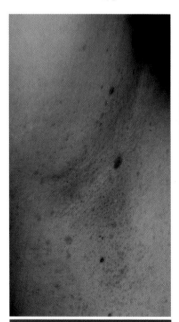

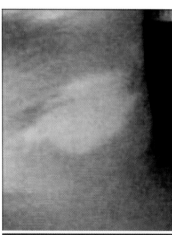

Figure 9-22: Ash leaf Hypopigmented

cardiac rhabdomyomas, but these regress over time. Another associated complication is infantile spasms, which, if they occur, indicate a 50% risk that tuberous sclerosis is present. The ash leaf hypopigmented macules usually enhance with a Woods lamp, and this can be helpful in diagnosis.

Tuberous sclerosis maps to either chromosome 9 or 16.

Most management is to deal with seizures or cardiac arrhythmias associated with the cardiac rhabdomyomas. Treat infantile spasms with vigabatrin.

CANCER GENETIC SYNDROMES

Familial cancer predisposing syndromes:
- Mendelian disorders
- Germline mutations
- Genes involved in familial cancer syndromes are also involved in sporadic tumors
- Involve proto-oncogenes, tumor suppressor genes, genes involved in DNA repair, apoptosis, integrity

Features of cancer syndromes:
- Family history
  ◦ Multiple members in family
- Early age of onset
- Bilateral/multifocal
- Clustering of specific types
  ◦ Breast and ovarian
  ◦ Retinoblastoma and osteosarcoma
- Multiple tumor types in same person
- Unusual type

von HIPPEL-LINDAU SYNDROME

von Hippel-Lindau (VHL) syndrome is a highly penetrant, AD multisystem cancer disorder that presents with various benign and malignant tumors of the eyes, CNS, kidneys, pancreas, adrenal glands, and reproductive adrenal glands. It occurs in about 1/36,000 live births.

It is caused by a mutation in the VHL tumor suppressor gene on chromosome 3. Molecular genetic testing of the *VHL* gene detects mutations in nearly 100% of patients.

Diagnosis depends on finding:
2 or more hemangioblastomas in the:
- CNS (particularly cerebellum), or
- retina;
Or, finding 1 single hemangioblastoma with either:
- pheochromocytoma,
- endolymphatic sac tumors,
- cysts in the kidney/pancreas,
- renal cell carcinoma, or
- pancreas involvement, neuroendocrine tumors;
Or, having a 1st degree relative and any 1 manifestation listed above.

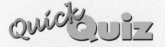

The most classic presentation is a cerebellar hemangioblastoma in adolescence or a retinal angioma by 10 years of age. Renal cysts are common. Renal cell carcinoma presents in the 40s and is the leading cause of mortality in VHL, occurring in nearly 40% of patients.

THE *PTEN* HAMARTOMA TUMOR SYNDROME

The *PTEN* hamartoma tumor syndrome (PHTS) includes Cowden syndrome (CS), Bannayan-Riley-Ruvalcaba syndrome (BRRS), Proteus syndrome (PS), and Proteus-like syndrome. CS is a multiple hamartoma syndrome with a high risk of benign and malignant tumors of the thyroid, breast, and endometrium. Affected individuals usually have macrocephaly, trichilemmomas, and papillomatous papules and present by the late 20s. The lifetime risk of developing breast cancer is 25–50%, with an average age of diagnosis between 38 and 46 years. The lifetime risk for thyroid cancer (usually follicular, rarely papillary, but never medullary thyroid cancer) is around 10%. The risk for endometrial cancer, although not well defined, may approach 5–10%. BRRS is a congenital disorder characterized by macrocephaly, intestinal hamartomatous polyposis, lipomas, and pigmented macules of the glans penis. PS is a complex, highly variable disorder involving congenital malformations and hamartomatous overgrowth of multiple tissues, as well as connective tissue nevi, epidermal nevi, and hyperostoses. Proteus-like syndrome is undefined but refers to individuals with significant clinical features of PS who do not meet the diagnostic criteria for PS.

Diagnosis/testing: The diagnosis of PHTS is made only when a *PTEN* mutation is identified. Approximately 85% of individuals who meet the diagnostic criteria for CS and 65% of individuals with a clinical diagnosis of BRRS have a detectable *PTEN* gene mutation.

TWO-HIT ORIGIN OF CANCER

Retinoblastoma is a good model of the "2-hit origin of cancer."
- Basis for both hereditary and sporadic cancers
- Involves loss of tumor suppressor function
- Retinoblastoma (RB) as the model
  - Loss of both copies of *RB1* gene leads to tumor
  - Sporadic cases: 2 somatic mutations in same cell
  - Hereditary cases: inherited (germline) mutation (first hit) and second somatic mutation in same cell (second hit)
- Loss of heterozygosity (LOH)
  - Molecular evidence for the existence of a tumor suppressor gene
  - Involves analysis of DNA polymorphisms near tumor suppressor genes
  - Test is done on tumor tissue

TERATOGENS

Thalidomide

Even today, thalidomide is a big Board exam question. It was one of the first drugs identified as a human teratogen. If fetal exposure occurs at 34–50 days of gestation, there is a 20% risk for limb defects, including missing arms and/or legs, and ear malformations with deafness. It was originally used as an anti-nausea drug but, as everyone now knows, has been pulled from the market for that indication in pregnancy. Now, it is marketed in the U.S. for treatment of peripheral neuropathies in Hansen disease, as well as HIV care. Obviously, a woman of childbearing potential should not use it.

Carbamazepine

Carbamazepine (Tegretol®) carries a < 1% risk of spina bifida when exposure occurs between days 15 and 29 after conception.

Methotrexate

Methotrexate, when taken between gestation weeks 6 and 9 at doses > 10 mg/week, can result in an increased risk of craniosynostosis, craniofacial abnormalities, and limb defects.

ACE Inhibitors

Use of ACE inhibitors during the 2nd and 3rd trimesters increases the risk of renal dysgenesis, oligohydramnios, and skull ossification defects.

Diethylstilbestrol (DES)

Diethylstilbestrol (DES) use before 12-weeks gestation increases the risk of vaginal adenocarcinoma developing in the offspring of the fetus at a later age. There also are reports of uterine abnormalities, vaginal adenosis, and male infertility.

notes

Lithium

Lithium use before 8-weeks gestation is associated with < 1% chance of Ebstein anomaly.

Phenytoin

Phenytoin use during the 1st trimester has a 10% risk of the fetal hydantoin syndrome (FHS: growth deficiency, developmental delays, craniofacial anomalies, hypoplastic phalanges/nails). There is also a 30% risk of having some of the adverse effects of FHS or vitamin K deficiency, resulting in bleeding problems.

Retinoic Acid

microtia =
small
ears

The agents of concern include isotretinoin, etretinate, and mega doses of vitamin A (retinol), which are used to treat acne and psoriasis. Highest risk periods of exposure are 2–5 weeks after conception, but exposure throughout pregnancy can cause serious malformations: findings similar to DiGeorge syndrome, microcephaly, facial nerve palsies, microtia and external auditory canal anomalies, cardiovascular defects, thymic hypoplasia, and genitourinary anomalies.

Streptomycin

Streptomycin use during the 3rd trimester is associated with hearing loss in the infant.

Tetracycline

Tetracycline use after 20-weeks gestation is associated with bone and tooth staining.

Valproic Acid

Valproic acid use in the first 30 days after conception has a 2% risk of spina bifida. Use during the 1st trimester can result in craniofacial abnormalities and preaxial defects.

Warfarin

Warfarin use during gestation weeks 6–9 can cause fetal warfarin syndrome, with nasal hypoplasia and stippled epiphyses. The overall risk approaches 30% of exposed pregnancies, and will result in fetal warfarin syndrome, CNS effects, or spontaneous abortions.

MATERNAL EXPOSURES AND ABUSES

Alcohol

Heavy use of alcohol (8–10 drinks or more/day) during pregnancy can result in a child with fetal alcohol syndrome; but as few as 2 drinks/day can lead to abnormal effects.

To diagnose, you must find the following in 3 distinct categories, along with substantiated maternal alcohol use:

1) Facial. Must have 2 of the following (see Figure 9-23):
   ◦ Shortened palpebral fissures
   ◦ Epicanthal folds
   ◦ Hypoplastic nasal root
   ◦ Short upturned nose
   ◦ Hypoplastic or absent philtrum
   ◦ Thin upper lip
   ◦ Midface hypoplasia

2) Pre- or postnatal growth deficiency. Must have 1:
   ◦ Weight < 10th percentile
   ◦ Microcephaly
   ◦ Length/height ratio < 10th percentile

3) Cognitive abnormality. Must have 1:
   ◦ Developmental or learning problems

Definitive diagnosis may not be made until the child is at least 4–8 years of age, because of changes in the facies. Also, non-European "norms" for short, upturned nose or midface hypoplasia are not well established.

Fetal alcohol syndrome is the most frequently documented cause of mental retardation.

Cigarette Smoking

Cigarette smoking has a high association with low birth weight. Recent data indicate that heavy cigarette smoking (> 10 cigarettes/day) can lead to miscarriage, prematurity, and stillbirth.

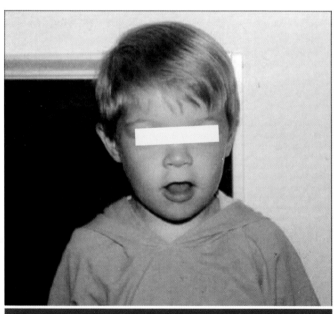

Figure 9-23: Fetal Alcohol Syndrome

notes

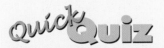

Cocaine

Cocaine use during pregnancy is associated with increased risk of miscarriage, stillbirth, and premature delivery. If used near delivery, cocaine can increase the risk of intracranial hemorrhage. Infants born to chronic users during pregnancy are frequently jittery, irritable, tremulous, and have muscle rigidity. These latter findings usually occur several days after birth and resolve quickly without known long-term effects.

Mercury (Fish Ingestion)

Mercury is an organic compound found in many fish products. If consumed during pregnancy, mercury poisoning in the fetus can manifest as cerebral atrophy, seizures, and developmental delay.

MATERNAL DISEASES

Diabetes Mellitus

Diabetes mellitus is the most common human teratogenic state! Mothers who require insulin during pregnancy have 2–3 times greater risk of having a child with a congenital defect. Defects can include sacral agenesis, situs abnormalities, holoprosencephaly, and congenital heart disease. It is important to get glucose levels under control before conception, which can markedly reduce the risk of congenital defects.

Hypertension

Hypertension occurring before the 20th week of gestation increases the risk of miscarriage. Hypertension occurring after the 20th week is associated with intrauterine growth restriction (IUGR), placental insufficiency, and placenta abruption or previa.

Hyperthermia
(Hot Tub Users and High Maternal Fever)

Extensive hyperthermia for prolonged periods during days 14–30 post-conception increases the risk of neural tube defects.

Systemic Lupus Erythematosus (SLE)

SLE is associated with an increased risk of spontaneous abortion in pregnancy before 20 weeks. After 20 weeks, it is associated with increased risk of stillbirth, prematurity, and congenital heart block.

MATERNAL INFECTIONS

Note

These are discussed in more detail in the Infectious Disease section.

Human Parvovirus B19 (Fifth Disease)

Infection with parvovirus B19 between weeks 10 and 24 of pregnancy can result in a 7–10% risk of the fetus developing congestive heart failure (hydrops) and dying.

Varicella

Varicella infection during the 1st trimester (8–20 weeks) results in a risk of fetal abnormalities in about 1–2%. Limb reduction defects can occur if the infection occurs prior to, or during, limb bud formation. Other effects you may see include chorioretinitis, skin scarring, developmental delay, and microcephaly.

Rubella

The frequency of fetal infection from mothers with rubella during the 1st trimester is ~ 50%.
Findings of congenital rubella syndrome depend on when the infection occurs:
• Up to 8 weeks: deafness (85% affected)
• 9–12 weeks: cataracts (52% affected)
• 12–30 weeks: heart defects (16% affected)

Cytomegalovirus (CMV)

CMV affects 5% of infants who are infected before the 27th week of gestation. Look for low birth weight, mental retardation, microcephaly, periventricular calcifications, and hearing loss that may not be present at birth but develop after the neonatal period.

Toxoplasmosis

Toxoplasmosis affects infants between weeks 10 and 24 of gestation and can present with hydrocephalus, blindness, and mental retardation.

Syphilis

Untreated syphilis can result in various abnormalities, particularly if infection occurs after 5 months gestation. The most commonly described findings are abnormal teeth and bones, mental retardation, and proteinuria.

notes

The following tables list commonly tested congenital anomaly syndromes. Review these well—especially if you are taking the initial certification exam.

Table 9-3: Commonly Tested Congenital Anomaly Syndromes 1

Craniofacial Syndromes		
Syndrome	Signs and Symptoms	Inheritance Pattern
Treacher-Collins syndrome	Cleft palate, malar hypoplasia, micrognathia, lower eyelid missing medial lower lid lashes, hearing loss	AD 100% *TCOF1* mut
Waardenburg syndrome I	Partial albinism, white forelock, premature graying, telecanthus (lateral displacement of inner canthi of eyes), heterochromia of iris, cleft lip/palate, cochlear deafness, occasional absent vagina, occasional Hirschsprung disease	AD > 90% *PAX3* mut
Stickler syndrome with Pierre Robin sequence	Micrognathia, cleft palate, glossoptosis (backward displacement of the tongue), airway obstruction, feeding difficulty, high myopia, retinal detachment	AD 70–80% *COL2A1* 70–80% *COL11A1*
Crouzon syndrome	Craniosynostosis with turricephaly, proptosis, hypertelorism, strabismus, maxillary hypoplasia	AD 100% *FGFR2* mut
Apert syndrome	Craniosynostosis, brachycephaly, acrocephaly, hypertelorism, proptosis, strabismus, maxillary hypoplasia, narrow palate ("cathedral ceiling"), syndactyly, "single nails," broad thumbs (most commonly with complete fusion of 2, 3, 4 fingers)	AD 100% *FGFR2* mut
Cleidocranial dysostosis	Brachycephaly, frontal bossing, wormian bones, delayed eruption of deciduous and permanent teeth, supernumerary and fused teeth, hypoplastic/absent clavicles, joint laxity	AD 60–70% *RUNX2* mut

Table 9-4: Commonly Tested Congenital Anomaly Syndromes 2

Chromosome Instability Syndromes		
Syndrome	Signs and Symptoms	Inheritance Pattern
Ataxia-telangiectasia	Ataxia, telangiectasia, frequent infections, malignancies, growth failure, worsening CNS function	AR > 95% *ATM* mut
Xeroderma pigmentosa	Photosensitivity, skin atrophy, pigmentary changes, malignancies	AR
Bloom syndrome	IUGR, microcephaly, malar hypoplasia, facial telangiectasia, malignancies	AR
Fanconi anemia	Pancytopenia, hypoplastic thumb and radius, hyperpigmentation, abnormal facial features	AR

notes

Table 9-5: Commonly Tested Congenital Anomaly Syndromes 3

Syndromes with Short Stature		
Syndrome	Signs and Symptoms	Inheritance Pattern
Cornelia De Lange syndrome	IUGR, microcephaly, hirsutism, down-turned mouth, heart defects micro-brachycephaly, micrognathia, low hairline, synophrys, long eyelashes, thin upper lip, "low-set ears," micromelia (hands/feet), or phocomelia; 2,3 syndactyly of toes	AD 50% have a gene mutation (*NIPBL*)
Dubowitz syndrome	IUGR, telecanthus, ptosis, eczema, hypotrichosis, behavioral and developmental disorders	AR
Noonan syndrome	Short stature, congenital heart defects (commonly pulmonary valve stenosis), pectus excavatum, webbed neck, hypertelorism, lymphedema, bleeding diathesis	AD ~ 50% *PTPN11* mut
Williams syndrome	Growth delay, mental retardation, stellate iris, hypoplastic nails, periorbital fullness, anteverted nares, supravalvular aortic stenosis	7q11 microdeletion

Table 9-6: Commonly Tested Congenital Anomaly Syndromes 4

Syndromes with Growth Abnormalities		
Syndrome	Signs and Symptoms	Inheritance Pattern
Prader-Willi syndrome (paternal)	Severe hypotonia at birth, obesity (usually after age 2 years), short stature, small hands and feet, hypogonadism, mild mental retardation	15q11–13 deletion, UPD
Angelman syndrome (maternal)	Jerky ataxic movements (the "happy puppet"), characteristic gait, hypotonia, fair hair, midface hypoplasia, prognathism, seizures, uncontrollable bouts of laughter, severe mental retardation	15q11–13 deletion, UPD, *UBE3A* mut
Sotos syndrome	LGA, macrocephaly, prominent forehead, hypertelorism, mental retardation, large hands/feet	AD 80–90% *NSD1* mut or deletion (5q35)
Beckwith-Wiedemann syndrome	Coarse facies, macroglossia, ear lobe creases, posterior auricular pits, omphalocele, Wilms tumor, cryptorchidism, hemihypertrophy	AD 11p15.5 deletion, UPD, multiple gene muts (*KCNQIOTI, H19, CKNIC*)
Proteus syndrome	Macrodactyly, soft tissue hypertrophy, hemihypertrophy, nevi, lipomas, lymphangiomata, hemangiomata, accelerated growth	Sporadic

notes

Table 9-7: Commonly Tested Congenital Anomaly Syndromes 5

Syndromes with Limb Abnormalities		
Syndrome	Signs and Symptoms	Inheritance Pattern
Möbius syndrome	Cranial nerve abnormalities, hypoplastic tongue and/or digits, limb deficiency, Poland anomaly (consisting of absence of the pectoralis major/minor muscles), ipsilateral breast hypoplasia (absence of two to four rib segments)	Sporadic
Rubinstein-Taybi syndrome	Short stature and limbs, microcephaly, beaked nose, broad thumbs and great toes, congenital heart disease, mental retardation	AD Microdeletion *CREBBP* mut 30–50%, FISH deletion ~10%, del/dup gene 10–20%

Table 9-8: Commonly Tested Congenital Anomaly Syndromes 6

Syndromes with Thumb/Radii Defects and Hematologic Abnormalities		
Syndrome	Signs and Symptoms	Inheritance Pattern
Fanconi anemia	Pancytopenia, hypoplastic thumb and radius, hyperpigmentation, abnormal facial features	AR
Diamond-Blackfan syndrome	Triphalangeal thumb, radial hypoplasia, hypoplastic anemia, congenital heart defects	AD
Thrombocytopenia-absent radius (TAR) syndrome	Thrombocytopenia, absent radii, normal thumbs, petechiae	AR
Holt-Oram syndrome	Radial ray abnormalities (triphalangeal thumb), ASD and other congenital heart disease	AD

notes

Table 9-9: Commonly Tested Congenital Anomaly Syndromes 7

Syndromes with Severe Neurologic Manifestations

Syndrome	Signs and Symptoms	Inheritance Pattern
Meckel-Gruber syndrome	Encephalocele (occipital), microcephaly, polycystic (dysplastic) kidney, polydactyly, lethal	AR
Miller-Dieker syndrome	Lissencephaly, microcephaly, micrognathia, anteverted nares, vertical wrinkles of the forehead	del 17p
Angelman/Prader-Willi syndrome	(See Table 9–6)	
Walker-Warburg (HARD + E) syndrome	Hydrocephalus, agyria (congenital lack of the convolutional pattern of the cerebral cortex), retinal dysplasia, encephalocele	AR
Sturge-Weber syndrome	Hemangioma in trigeminal nerve distribution, glaucoma, seizures, meningeal hemangiomata	Sporadic
Rett syndrome	Normal psychomotor development ~ 6–18 months, followed by rapid regression in language and motor skills; repetitive, stereotypic hand movements replace purposeful hand use; autistic features; episodic apnea and/or hyperpnea; gait ataxia; tremors; seizures; and acquired microcephaly	80% *MeCP2* mut, 8% deletion/duplication

Table 9-10: Commonly Tested Congenital Anomaly Syndromes 8

Metabolic Syndromes with Congenital Anomalies
(Discussed in the Metabolic Disorders section)

Syndrome	Signs and Symptoms	Inheritance Pattern
Menkes syndrome	Progressive neurologic deterioration, sparse and broken hair (pili torti), skeletal changes, decreased serum copper and ceruloplasmin	X-linked
Zellweger syndrome	Hypotonia, flat occiput, epicanthal folds, hepatomegaly, camptodactyly (flexion of one or both interphalangeal joints of one or more fingers, usually the little finger), cerebral defects, retinal lesions, renal cysts, peroxisomal defects	AR
Glutaric acidemia Type II	Hepatomegaly, facial dysmorphism, renal cysts, GU anomalies	AR
Smith-Lemli-Opitz syndrome	Short stature, microcephaly, ptosis, anteverted nares, syndactyly of toes 2, 3; cryptorchidism, hypospadias, mental retardation, cholesterol metabolism defect	AR
Wilson disease	Kayser-Fleisher rings, abnormal copper metabolism	AR
Kallmann syndrome	Short stature, mental retardation, hypogonadotropic hypogonadism, anosmia	X-linked

notes

Table 9-11: Commonly Tested Congenital Anomaly Syndromes 9

Common Associations and Other Miscellaneous Syndromes

Syndrome	Signs and Symptoms	Inheritance Pattern
VATER/VACTERL	Vertebral defects, anal atresia, tracheoesophageal fistula, radial dysplasia, renal malformations, congenital heart defect	Sporadic
CHARGE	Coloboma, congenital heart defects, choanal atresia, growth and mental retardation, GU anomalies (hypogonadism), ear anomaly	*CHD7* on Chr 8q
MURCS	Müllerian duct aplasia, renal aplasia, cervicothoracic somite dysplasia	Sporadic
Opitz syndrome (GBB syndrome)	Hypertelorism, telecanthus, high nasal bridge, cleft lip/palate, hypospadias, laryngotracheoesophageal cleft	XD/AD
McCune-Albright syndrome	Multiple bony fibrous dysplasia, "café-au-lait" spots, sexual precocity	Sporadic
Alagille syndrome	Bile duct paucity with cholestasis, pulmonary artery stenosis, posterior embryotoxon, butterfly vertebrae, characteristic triangular-shaped facies with long nose, broad mid-nose, and pointed chin	AD 2 genes, 88% *JAG1* mut, 7% FISH deletion of *JAG1* on 20p12, <1% *NOTCH2* mut
Neurofibromatosis, Type 1	Macrocephaly, neurofibroma, plexiform neurofibroma, dysplasia of the sphenoid bone, malignancies (< 5%), learning disability, optic glioma, Lisch nodules	AD Neurofibromin (17p) gene

MedStudy®

4th Edition

Pediatrics Board Review Core Curriculum

Metabolic Disorders

Authored by J. Thomas Cross, Jr., MD, MPH, FAAP, and Robert A. Hannaman, MD

Many thanks to

Sara Copeland, MD
Clinical Assistant Professor in Pediatrics
Division of Medical Genetics / Department of Pediatrics
University of Iowa Hospitals and Clinics
Medical Director, Iowa Neonatal Metabolic Screening
Iowa City, IA

Metabolic Disorders Advisor

INTOXICATIONS

Overview

Symptoms result from upstream buildup of chemicals that cause symptoms because of toxicity to other cells.
They present in several forms:
- Acute encephalopathy
- Chronic encephalopathy
- Acid-base disturbances

Examples include:
- Amino acid disorders
- Urea cycle defects
- Organic acidurias

Acute Encephalopathy Presentation

Suspect inborn errors if acute encephalopathy occurs in neonates or young infants—or occurs suddenly without warning and progresses rapidly.
Symptoms can include:
- Unexplained seizures
- Coma
- Lethargy
- Hypertonia
- Hypotonia

Because of the acute onset, it is usually not associated with focal neurologic deficits. Often, there is a history of some form of stress, fasting, illness, or increased protein load. Most of these diseases are due to small molecules, specifically those that are water-soluble and easily get into the brain, such as glucose, ammonia, and amino and organic acids.
Examples of the more common, associated diseases are:
- maple syrup urine disease,
- ornithine transcarbamoylase (OTC) deficiency, and
- propionic acidemia.

Most of these infants are normal at birth and their mothers had a normal pregnancy. However, once the maternal circulation is removed, the ability of the infant to handle the extra substrates or metabolites is compromised. Thus, you get large increases in brain-diffusible substrate or metabolite that causes toxic effects on the brain. The infant begins to have feeding problems, lethargy, irritability, and vomiting. Commonly, the metabolic inequities will be much more pronounced when the infant/child is under stress or in an increased catabolic state (such as with viral/bacterial illness).

Generally, 4 categories of "small molecule disease" will present with acute encephalopathy. Table 10-1 outlines key things to

look for on Board questions. Each will be discussed in more detail later in the chapter.

Once you identify these infants, work quickly to prevent further damage. The key is to provide adequate calories and hydration; most use 10% dextrose in 0.45% saline, with 20 mEq/L of potassium (if urine output is adequate), to run at 1.5x maintenance. You can give sodium bicarbonate if the serum bicarbonate level is < 15 mEq/L, but be careful not to overcorrect. You can use hemodialysis or hemofiltration to remove the small molecule that is causing the problem. Once you identify the specific problem, proceed with appropriate therapy.

Chronic Encephalopathy Presentation

Chronic encephalopathy presents as slowly progressive symptoms from the buildup of toxic metabolites. The symptoms are not sudden, nor are they immediately life-threatening. However, this may change over time as more and more damage occurs.

The most striking examples are phenylketonuria (PKU) and homocystinuria. Both of these cause symptoms after a period of exposure. With PKU, the buildup of phenylalanine eventually kills brain cells, causing loss of developmental milestones and eventually permanent brain damage. Homocystinuria causes problems after exposure to high levels of homocysteine and damage to the blood vessels, resulting in clots and stroke.

Acid-base Disturbances

Causes

This is generally due to one of two factors:
1) accumulation of fixed anions, or
2) loss of bicarbonate (this is almost always due to renal tubular dysfunction).

Table 10-1: Inborn Errors of Metabolism Presenting as Intoxications	
Disorder	Main lab to look for in the question
Amino acid diseases (Maple syrup urine)	Plasma amino and urine organic acids Metabolic acidosis with urine ketones Increased anion gap
Hyperammonemias (Ornithine transcarbamylase or OTC deficiency)	Plasma ammonium Minimal metabolic acidosis Respiratory alkalosis
Organic acid diseases (Propionic acidemia)	Metabolic acidosis with urine ketones Plasma ammonium Increased glycine Abnormal urine organic acids Increased anion gap
Sugar intolerances: galactosemia, fructose intolerance	Newborn screening enzymatic testing Urine organic acids Liver enzyme analysis

notes

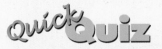

Accumulation of Fixed Anions

In this case, the plasma chloride concentration is normal, and the anion gap is increased > 13. These disorders become more pronounced in increased catabolic states, such as after surgery, with illness, or from changes in diet with increased protein intake. The child commonly presents with feeding difficulties and failure to thrive. The categories of disease include organic acidurias, ketoacidosis, and lactic acidosis +/– pyruvate elevations.

Loss of Bicarbonate

This is usually due to increased renal loss of bicarbonate secondary to renal injury. Proximal renal tubular dysfunction with loss of bicarbonate encompasses only a few disorders.

ENERGY DEFECTS

Overview

These disorders have symptoms related to the inability to use or make energy. Our bodies get energy during fasting, in a specific order. First, glucose in the blood, then breakdown of stored glycogen, then fatty acid oxidation, and, finally, breakdown of amino acids for making glucose. Therefore,

difficulties in any of these metabolites can cause problems. Disorders of energy metabolism can occur anywhere in the ATP pathway. Examples of these disorders are (see Table 10-2):
- fatty acid oxidation defects,
- glycogen storage diseases: defects making or breaking down glycogen,
- Krebs cycle/mitochondrial respiratory chain disorders, including the congenital lactic acidosis.

Presentation

Fasting or illness with increased energy needs can exacerbate the disorder and bring on decompensation. There may or may not be hypoglycemia. Patients may present with failure to thrive, hypotonia, cardiac dysfunction, lactic acidosis, or weakness and fatigue. The presentation is determined by the effect on the cells. If muscle is affected, such as with mitochondrial defects, then weakness is a symptom. If the body is unable to utilize the oxidative phosphorylation pathway, lactic acid will build up.

COMPLEX MOLECULE DEFECTS

Overview

These are chronic progressive disorders. They are generally not present at birth but may be evident in infancy if the enzyme defect is severe enough. When congenital in onset, the most common feature is hydrops. Features are secondary to buildup in cells of large molecules that cause cellular dysfunction and even death. (See Table 10-3.)

Presentation is usually 1 of 3 forms:
1) Dysmorphic/coarse features syndromes
2) Severe bone dysplasia
3) Neurological presentation
   ◦ Seizures
   ◦ Loss of skills
   ◦ Deafness
   ◦ Blindness
   ◦ Learning problems
   ◦ Behavior problems
   ◦ Early onset dementia
   ◦ Abnormal tone

These are rare and difficult to "tease out" in the diagnosis. The most commonly seen on Boards are:
- Hurler disease
- Hunter disease
- Albinism
- Mevalonic aciduria
- PDH deficiency
- Zellweger syndrome
- Infantile G_{m1}-gangliosidosis
- Familial hypercholesterolemia

Table 10-2: Presentation of Various Disorders of Energy Metabolism	
Fatty acid oxidation defects	Hypoketotic hypoglycemia Hypotonia Cardiomyopathy SIDS death
Glycogen storage diseases	Hepatomegaly Hypoglycemia Lactic acidosis Failure to thrive
Mitochondrial disorders	Lactic acidosis Seizures Cardiomyopathy Hypotonia/myopathy +/– hypoglycemia

notes

Lysosomal Disorders

Lysosomal diseases make sense. Either you have an enzyme defect, where the macromolecules in the lysosome can't break down, or, once you break down the molecule, the lysosome can't ship it out (efflux problems). Cell death occurs when the lysosome either can't digest the bad molecule or can't send it out of the cell once it is digested. The major macromolecules the lysosome has to deal with are the glycosaminoglycans, glycoproteins, gangliosides, and glycolipids. So you will see problems occur only in those body cells and tissues where the lysosomes are disturbed!

Peroxisomal Disorders

Peroxisomes are responsible for bile acid; plasmalogen synthesis and oxidation of very long-chain fatty acids; phytanic acid; and pipecolic acid. The key feature of peroxisomal diseases is severe, progressive CNS dysfunction, usually starting in infancy. All of these functions are important to neuronal development, structure, and function.

Other key items to look for in Board questions:
- Facial dysmorphism
- Eye findings
- Brain migrational defects with abnormal MRI findings
- Hepatomegaly with liver dysfunction
- Renal cysts
- Hypotonia

All of the peroxisomal disorders are AR (except X-linked adrenoleukodystrophy).

Intracellular Trafficking and Processing

These disorders are difficult to demonstrate because their symptoms are often multi-organ. Their diagnosis depends on the measurement of plasma levels of specific proteins, such as α-antitrypsin, glycosylated transferrin, thyroid-binding globulin, or total serum glycoproteins.

Inborn Errors of Cholesterol Synthesis

These disorders occur anywhere in the biosynthesis of cholesterol or its downstream metabolites. They have a wide spectrum of symptoms, ranging from high cholesterol and early heart disease, to problems with myelin formation and neurological symptoms, to bile acid synthesis defects and subsequent disorders in digestion.

DISORDERS OF AMINO ACID METABOLISM
OVERVIEW

The most valuable diagnostic tests are examination of plasma amino acids and urine organic acids. You need to do both. These disorders are typically single-gene deficiencies. Systemic manifestations are common because of the large amount of small molecule metabolites in the circulation, frequently resulting in mental retardation. These disorders fall into the intoxication classification of disorders. Presentation may be either acute or chronic depending on the disorder.

Table 10-3: Complex Molecule Defects	
Lysosomal storage diseases	Mucopolysaccharidoses (MPS) types I–IX Gaucher disease Niemann-Pick disease, types A, B, C Tay-Sachs disease Fabry disease Neuronal ceroid lipofuscinosis
Peroxisomal storage diseases	Zellweger syndrome spectrum X-linked adrenoleukodystrophy (X-ALD) Refsum disease Mevalonate kinase Rhizomelic chondrodysplasia punctata
Intracellular trafficking and processing defects	Menkes disease (kinky hair disease, copper defect) Wilson disease (copper defect) Hemochromatosis (iron defect) Alpha-1-antitrypsin deficiency Congenital disorders of glycosylation
Inborn errors of cholesterol synthesis	Smith-Lemli-Opitz syndrome Hypercholesterolemia, autosomal dominant Apolipoprotein E deficiency Tangier disease Desmosterolosis

PHENYLALANINE-TYROSINE DISORDERS

Classic Phenylketonuria (PKU)

PKU is an AR disorder in which phenylalanine cannot be converted to tyrosine. The enzyme defect is in phenylalanine hydroxylase (PAH). This results in high levels of phenylalanine in the blood and large amounts of phenylpyruvic acid in the urine. PKU occurs in 1/10,000 to 1/20,000 births. The gene for phenylalanine hydroxylase is carried on chromosome 12q24.1.

Clinical findings vary, depending on when treatment is initiated and on the degree of metabolic control. Phenylalanine in high amounts is toxic to the CNS. Those who remain untreated have severe mental retardation with IQs of < 30. The damage becomes irreversible by age 8 weeks. PKU infants appear normal at birth, but early symptoms occur in > 50% of those affected. The most common presentations in infants include vomiting, irritability, an eczematoid rash, and a peculiar odor—"mousy,"

notes

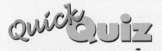
"wolf-like," or musty in character—which is due to the phenylacetic acid in the urine. Nearly all of those affected are fair-haired and fair-skinned, compared to their unaffected relatives. EEGs are abnormal.

You must make the diagnosis in the neonatal period to prevent serious consequences. In the U.S., universal newborn screening for PKU in the first few days of life occurs in all 50 states. If a positive screen occurs, next is a quantitative analysis of the concentrations of phenylalanine and tyrosine.

Most patients identified by the screening test are false-positives due to delayed maturation of amino acid-metabolizing enzymes and very high tyrosine concentrations. About 1–2% of patients with hyperphenylalaninemia will not have a defect in phenylalanine hydroxylase and instead will have a problem with synthesis or recycling of biopterin.

Therapy is straightforward if not easy: limit the dietary intake of phenylalanine. All infants should be supervised by a dietician familiar with PKU, and Phe levels should be frequently monitored to see how much dietary restriction is necessary. You must give phenylalanine for normal growth and development, even in PKU infants. All patients with PKU should stay on the special diet for life. Even after infancy, CNS damage occurs if the Phe levels are allowed to get too high.

Maternal PKU refers to the teratogenic effects of elevated phenylalanine on the developing fetus in a mother with untreated PKU. Infants do not actually have PKU but may have growth deficiency, microcephaly, mental retardation, and congenital heart defects—very similar to fetal alcohol syndrome.

Hyperphenylalaninemia

These are patients without classic PKU but who have elevated levels of phenylalanine in the blood. These infants will generally tolerate higher levels of dietary phenylalanine. But this depends on the individual.

A subset of these patients, however, comprises those with a defect in the synthesis or recycling of biopterin. These patients will have neurologic symptoms that progress in spite of dietary treatment that maintains normal phenylalanine levels. They have a defect in either the synthesis of tetrahydro-biopterin, a cofactor for phenylalanine hydroxylase, or they have a defect in the enzymes that regenerate tetrahydrobiopterin from dihydrobiopterin. Both of these will result in diminished conversion of phenylalanine to tyrosine. Tetrahydrobiopterin is also a cofactor for the hydroxylation of tryptophan and tyrosine, so you get interference in synthesis of important compounds, such as serotonin, dopa, and norepinephrine.

Clinically these infants present with severe neurologic disease with marked hypotonia, spasticity, and posturing. Drooling is common, and psychomotor developmental delay is marked.

Treatment includes phenylalanine restriction and biopterin supplementation, as well as giving them biogenic amine precursors, such as 5-hydroxytryptophan and dopa.

Tyrosinemia

Tyrosinemia refers to a group of disorders with a common theme of elevated tyrosine levels in body fluids. The most common form, particularly in premature infants, is a "transient" tyrosinemia due to delayed maturation of tyrosine-metabolizing enzymes. Tyrosinemia can occur in scurvy and liver diseases. We will discuss the 3 more common genetic deficiencies of enzymes here; they all are AR.

Hereditary tyrosinemia Type I (tyrosinosis, hepatorenal tyrosinemia) is due to a deficiency of fumarylacetoacetate hydroxylase, which is the final step in tyrosine metabolism. Symptoms result from accumulation of the succinylacetone; the tyrosine is a marker for the disease, but not the damaging end product.

Infants are affected early, and most have a rapid course to death; some, however, progress more slowly. FTT and hepatomegaly with hepatoblastoma are the most common presentations. These infants are not mentally retarded. They have renal tubular acidosis resembling Fanconi syndrome, as well as x-ray findings of rickets.

You can diagnose this type by finding elevated levels of tyrosine in the plasma, but the definitive diagnostic finding is succinylacetone in the urine.

You can treat liver failure and Fanconi syndrome of hepatorenal tyrosinemia with 2-(nitro-4-trifuoro-methyl-benzolyl)-1,3-cyclohexanedione, also known (thank goodness) as NTBC. This blocks tyrosine metabolism before the fumarylacetoacetate hydroxylase enzyme, which prevents the accumulation of toxic metabolites. Since NTBC blocks tyrosine breakdown, tyrosine levels are elevated, causing secondary tyrosinemia with symptoms like tyrosinemia Type II if not treated. Patients must be on a diet low in tyrosine and phenylalanine.

Tyrosinemia Type II (Richner-Hanhart syndrome, oculocutaneous tyrosinemia) is a deficiency of tyrosine aminotransferase, which is the first step of tyrosine metabolism. Patients present with corneal ulcers or dendritic keratitis, along with red papular or keratotic lesions on their palms and soles. 50% will have mental retardation. They do not have the liver toxicity seen in Type I disease since they do not build up succinylacetone. The eye and skin lesions are from deposition of tyrosine itself. Treat with a diet low in tyrosine, but even this may not be curative.

Tyrosinemia Type III is very rare (so rare that only 4 cases have been reported, according to one source. Which reminds me—if you are pressed for time or can't stand this stuff, be sure you do know the yellow highlighted areas!). It is due to deficiency of 4-hydroxyphenypyruvate dioxygenase, and patients can have mental retardation. Patients respond well to a diet low in tyrosine.

Alkaptonuria

Alkaptonuria is due to deficiency in homogentisic acid dioxygenase, which is the 3rd step in tyrosine metabolism. However, blood levels of tyrosine are not elevated. Excretion of dark-colored urine is the classic finding in alkaptonuria.

This is an interesting syndrome. Fresh urine is normal but, as it "sits" and alkalinizes, the oxidation of homogentisic acid proceeds, and a dark-brown/black pigment forms—may be noted by parents in diapers, looking like brick dust. (Wow, what a great party trick.)

Most of these kids are asymptomatic. This disorder doesn't show up until adulthood, when they get a urinalysis for some other reason and their sample sits at the nursing station forever. By the time they are in their 30s, adults will start to have pigment deposition in the ears and sclerae. This is called ochronosis. Later, ochronosis arthritis can occur.

Infantile Parkinsonism

This is an AR deficiency of tyrosine hydroxylase and causes severe parkinsonism in infants. A less severe form of the disease is known as Segawa syndrome (dopa-responsive dystonia). Patients present between ages 1 and 9 years with dystonic posture or movement of one limb. Intelligence is normal. There is also an AD variant.

BRANCHED-CHAIN AMINO ACID DEFECTS

Cause/Diagnosis

The branched-chain amino acids (in case you forgot) are valine, leucine, and isoleucine. Problems in the breakdown of these 3 cause the accumulation of organic acid intermediates, resulting in toxic effects on various organ systems. Diagnose with urine organic acid test. Look for (smell for) a weird urine odor. AR inheritance is most common for these defects.

Maple Syrup Urine Disease

Classic maple syrup urine disease (MSUD) presents with CNS disease early in infancy, and the urine (or hair or skin) smells like maple syrup. Infants are well at birth but start having symptoms by 3–5 days of life, with rapid progression to death in 2–4 weeks without treatment. Babies have feeding difficulties, irregular respirations, or loss of the Moro reflex. Severe seizures, opisthotonos, and rigidity are common presenting signs. Death follows decerebrate rigidity from cerebral edema. Also, milder forms of the disease occur with intermittent, branched-chain aminoaciduria, characterized by ataxia and repeated episodes of lethargy, progressing to coma but without mental retardation. Stressors, such as infection, frequently induce this form.

The defect is in the oxidative decarboxylation of ketoacids (the ketoacids are what smell sweet), which are formed by catabolism of the branched-amino acids. AR mutations can occur in 4 different genes and cause MSUD. The incidence is ~ 1/150,000.

Determine diagnosis by finding increased amounts of leucine, isoleucine, and valine in the plasma and urine. Finding alloisoleucine, an abnormal amino acid, is diagnostic for MSUD.

Aim therapy at dietary control of leucine, isoleucine, and valine. If therapy is started early, before damage has occurred, normal IQ is possible. There is a very rare form of MSUD that responds very well to thiamine.

LYSINE, HYDROXYLYSINE, AND TRYPTOPHAN GROUP

Glutaric aciduria Type 1, an AR enzyme defect (glutaryl-CoA dehydrogenase) in the catabolic pathway of lysine, hydroxylysine, and tryptophan, is the only clinically relevant disorder in this group.

These infants present with macrocephaly at birth but generally have normal development until they have a febrile illness or metabolic stressor, when they suddenly develop hypotonia and dystonia.

CT/MRI shows frontal and cortical atrophy at birth with increased extra axial space and, after symptoms of dystonia develop, degeneration of the caudate nucleus and putamen occurs. Striatal degeneration occurs in some during the first few years of life if they have a metabolic decompensation. Diagnostically, urine organic acids will show increased excretion of glutaric and 3-hydroxyglutaric acids. Carnitine levels are usually low. The gene encoding glutaryl-CoA dehydrogenase is on chromosome 19. Treat with L-carnitine, riboflavin, and special diet—and rapid implementation of IV fluids containing glucose when ill, particularly with febrile illnesses. This regimen may prevent symptoms and striatal degeneration if given early, before symptoms develop. Five percent of patients will never have problems, and 35% of patients will have severe disease even with optimal therapy. This is the one metabolic disease that can cause subdural hematomas and retinal hemorrhages, which can be mistaken for child abuse. The increased extra axial space causes stretching of the bridging veins, making them susceptible to hematomas.

notes

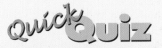

Quick Quiz

1) What is alkaptonuria? What is the "great party trick" these children can do?
2) What are the branched-chain amino acids?
3) Describe the symptoms of maple syrup urine disease.
4) How do you diagnose maple syrup urine disease?
5) Differentiate the lens findings in Marfan syndrome versus homocystinuria.
6) What molecule is "the problem" in all of the urea cycle disorders?

SULFUR-CONTAINING AMINO ACID DEFECTS

Homocystinuria

Homocystinuria is really a heterogeneous group of disorders caused by 6 types of genetic defects. Classically, the term was used specifically to indicate disease due to a defect in the cystathionine β-synthetase enzyme. This is an AR disorder found on chromosome 21q. All of the diseases in this group cause elevated levels of homocysteine. B_{12} metabolism defects can also cause homocysteine levels to rise.

Clinically, patients with cystathionine β-synthetase deficiency have marfanoid habitus, developmental delay, lens dislocation, and an increased risk of thromboembolism in both arteries and veins. With the exception of the embolisms, these symptoms may present within the first 10 years. The risk of embolic events persists into adult life. Clotting studies are normal, but elevated homocysteine levels cause increased platelet stickiness. On the Board exam, look for someone with subluxation/dislocation of the ocular lens, which is the most characteristic feature in real-life. Mental retardation is

fairly common. The joints are limited in mobility (not hypermobile as in Marfan syndrome) and also have osteoporosis. Lenticular subluxation is usually downward and medial. Memory aid: think of (downward = low IQ), as opposed to Marfan syndrome, which is upward (upward = normal IQ).

Large doses of pyridoxine may cause a decrease in the total plasma homocysteine levels (in the vitamin-responsive form). Generally they also require a diet low in methionine, the step feeding into homocysteine. These patients need to be followed by a metabolic specialist over time; betaine is another therapy that increases the conversion of homocysteine to methionine.

GLYCINE AND OXALATE ABNORMALITIES

Nonketotic Hyperglycinemia

This is an AR inborn error of metabolism, where you have large amounts of glycine in body fluids without detectable accumulation of organic acids. The highest levels of glycine are in the CNS. This presents as intractable seizures in the neonatal period or as hiccups *in utero* in the classic form. It may present as seizures and hypotonia in the milder, later-onset form of the disease. Severe mental retardation is common in those who survive. Diagnosis is made by looking at the ratio of glycine in the serum compared to that in the CSF. Prenatal diagnosis is possible by biochemical analysis of chorionic villus biopsy. Sodium benzoate seems to reduce CSF glycine levels and decrease seizures. Dextromethorphan also has been used with some success.

DISORDERS OF THE UREA CYCLE

The complete urea cycle (see Figure 10-1) occurs in the liver, specifically the periportal hepatocytes, and most of it occurs in the mitochondria. This cycle is responsible for removing nitrogen waste from the body. Ammonia (NH_4^+) is the problem here, and it is normally broken down initially into glycine, glutamine, and carbamyl phosphate via different enzymes. A cascade then follows: Carbamyl phosphate further breaks down into citrulline, which then breaks down into argininosuccinate, then arginine, and finally, the excretal urea into urine.

These fall into the intoxication classification of disorders. Presentation may be either acute or chronic depending on the disorder. However, all are prone to acute decompensations.

6 main enzyme defects can result in hyperammonemias due to urea cycle defects:
- N-acetylglutamate synthetase deficiency (NAGS deficiency)
- Carbamoyl phosphate synthetase 1 (CPS deficiency)
- Ornithine transcarbamoylase deficiency (OTC; most common and X-linked)
- Argininosuccinate synthetase deficiency (citrullinemia)

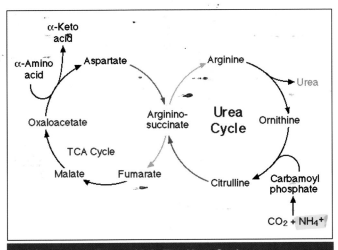

Figure 10-1: The Urea Cycle

notes

- Argininosuccinate lyase deficiency (argininosuccinic aciduria)
- Arginase deficiency (argininemia)

Also, there are 2 transport defects possible in the urea cycle that can cause hyperammonemias:

1) amino acid transporter gene *SLC7A7* (lysinuric protein intolerance or LPI); and
2) mitochondrial ornithine transporter *ORNT1* (HHH syndrome: hyperornithinemia, hyperammonemia, homocitrullinuria).

All of the urea cycle disorders, except for OTC deficiency, which has X-linked inheritance (and is most common), have autosomal recessive inheritance.

Ammonia and elevated CSF glutamine are significant problems because they have a toxic effect almost exclusively on the brain. Brain edema occurs quickly, and ammonia levels between 100 and 200 µmol/L will cause lethargy, vomiting, and confusion. Higher levels will result in coma.

Does it matter where the defect is in the cycle? Yes! Usually, the more proximal the defect is, the more severe the symptoms. Note: all defects have milder forms that may present later in life. The most severe are carbamoyl phosphate synthetase deficiency (CPS) and OTC deficiency. These infants are usually born normal and at term (because the mom can filter out the excess ammonia easily during pregnancy). But by 5 days of age, in the classic form of the disease, the elevated ammonia levels result in clinical symptoms of lethargy, hypotonia, vomiting, and poor feeding. These children progress rapidly to coma and death if the hyperammonemia is not quickly identified and treated. Plasma ammonia levels can be > 1,000 µmol/L (normal < 35). A key diagnostic clue on the Boards is if they mention a blood gas! These infants usually have a respiratory alkalosis, not a

metabolic acidosis, as you would expect with sepsis.

Late-onset urea cycle defects do occur and usually are partial enzyme deficiencies, precipitated by infection or some other stressor. Females with OTC deficiency are a good example of later onset; their symptoms sometimes will be precipitated by pregnancy and childbirth.

Table 10-4 lists a few specific clinical abnormalities associated with some of the non-classic urea cycle defects. If they are present, consider it a clue!

When to think of urea cycle defects? On the Board exam, look for an elevated plasma ammonia in association with mild or no liver dysfunction and no ketoacidosis. Frequently, another clue will be a low BUN and respiratory alkalosis (not metabolic acidosis). Be aware that a precipitating event, such as infection or injury, is likely. Also be aware that valproate and haloperidol can "unmask" urea cycle defects.

Once you determine the child has a urea cycle defect, order quantitative plasma and urinary organic acids to establish the specific defect in urea synthesis. Glutamine, alanine, and asparagine will be elevated—because they are storage forms for nitrogen, which cannot be excreted. Plasma arginine concentration is always low in urea cycle defects, except in argininemia. To help determine if it is a proximal or a distal defect, order a citrulline level. It is absent or very low in disorders occurring proximally, such as in OTC and CPS defects, because citrulline is the product of these reactions. To differentiate between OTC and CPS, check a urinary orotic acid level. It will be elevated in OTC deficiency and normal/low in CPS and NAGS.

Treatment generally centers on restricting dietary nitrogen, replacing deficient amino acids, and pushing alternate pathways to eliminate nitrogen waste. Specifically, arginine is deficient in all disorders except for argininemia. Without replacement, affected individuals will have hair fragility and rash. The alternate pathways use sodium benzoate. This is conjugated in the liver with glycine and makes hippuric acid and sodium-phenylacetate, which is then conjugated with glutamine to form phenylacetylglutamine. The hippuric acid and phenylacetylglutamine will be easily excreted in the urine. If the plasma ammonia level is > 200 µmol/L and/or the infant is in a coma, hemodialysis is the only way to clear the ammonia. Chronic management involves a high-caloric, protein-restricted diet with or without additional amino acids. More and more patients with infantile onset disease are having liver transplants with improved long-term outcomes.

ORGANIC ACIDEMIAS FROM AMINO ACID DISORDERS

OVERVIEW

Organic acidemias are characterized by urinary excretion of abnormal amounts or types of organic acids. An organic acid is a chemical compound with one or more carboxyl radicals (COOH) in its structure. These are inherited deficiencies in specific enzymes involved in the breakdown of

Table 10-4: Clinical Findings in Patients with Urea Cycle Defects	
Disorder	**Clinical Finding**
Argininemia	Progressive spastic diplegia/quadriplegia Tremor, ataxia, and choreoathetosis
HHH *Hyperornithemia Hyperammonemia Homocitrullinemia*	Progressive spastic diplegia/quadriplegia Retinal depigmentation Chorioretinal thinning
LPI	Interstitial pneumonia (due to pulmonary alveolar proteinosis) Glomerulonephritis Osteoporosis Underlying immune deficiency
Argininosuccinic aciduria	Trichorrhexis nodosa (node-like appearance of fragile hair) Episodic coma

notes

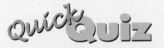

Quick Quiz

1) How are almost all urea cycle disorders inherited?
2) You are presented an infant with elevated ammonia, no liver abnormalities, and no ketoacidosis. What type of defect should you consider?
3) What is the importance of a citrulline level?
4) What is the importance of ordering a urinary orotic-acid level?
5) An infant with encephalopathy presents with a smell of "sweaty feet." What is a possible diagnosis?
6) How does propionic acidemia present in early infancy?
7) What is the triad of symptoms associated with carboxylase deficiency?

branched-chain amino acids, lysine, tryptophan, or fatty acids. They fall into the intoxication category of inborn errors of metabolism.

- In these disorders, the child gets a buildup of acids, which causes an anion gap metabolic acidosis with normal chloride. They are for the most part AR disorders.
- The kidneys clear most organic acids, so it is easiest to examine the urine for these disorders. All of these disorders have overlap in complications, including bone marrow suppression and pancreatitis.

ISOVALERIC ACIDEMIA

If you see the words "odor of sweaty feet," don't think of the boys' locker room but, rather, of isovaleric acidemia, especially if the question refers to an infant with encephalopathy. This is an AR disorder localized to chromosome 15 and is due to a defect in isovaleryl-CoA dehydrogenase. You can't convert isovaleryl-CoA to 3-methylcrotonyl-CoA, so you get increased levels of isovaleryl-CoA!

Isovaleric acidemia (IVA) can present in the newborn with an acute episode of severe metabolic acidosis and moderate ketosis with vomiting, which may lead to coma and death; but, more commonly, it presents in infancy or childhood and is precipitated by an infection or increased protein intake. A chronic intermittent form with pancytopenia and acidosis occurs in infants who survive the acute episode. Urine organic acids can be diagnostic of IVA by elevations of specific analytes. Prenatal diagnosis is possible.

Aim acute treatment at the acidosis, which will usually respond to IV glucose and bicarbonate. Center long-term treatment on restricting leucine intake and prescribing carnitine and/or glycine to increase conversion of isovaleryl-CoA to isovaleryl glycine, which can be excreted easily.

3-METHYLCROTONYL-CoA CARBOXYLASE DEFICIENCY

This is an AR disorder where the biotin-containing enzyme, 3-methylcrotonyl-CoA carboxylase (MCC), is missing and 3-methylcrotonyl-CoA is not converted to 3-methylglutaconyl-CoA.

Patients may present between ages 1 and 3 years with acute metabolic acidosis, hypoglycemia, and carnitine deficiency—usually during a stressor event; e.g., an infection. The majority probably will never have any decompensation or symptoms related to the enzyme defect. Urine organic acid analysis shows increased excretion of 3-methyl-crotonylglycine and 3-hydroxyisovaleric acid. Gear acute treatment toward IV glucose, fluids, and electrolytes. Aim long-term therapy at oral carnitine to correct carnitine deficiency, if present, and biotin to enhance enzymatic function. Those affected may never be ill and may be identified only when they have an abnormal newborn screen.

At this time, we cannot say who will have problems and who will not, so treat them all. Biotin may be helpful, so some are using it.

PROPIONIC ACIDEMIA

Propionic acidemia occurs as an AR disorder due to a deficiency in propionyl-CoA carboxylase (PCC), a biotin-containing enzyme that converts propionyl-CoA to D-methylmalonyl-CoA. Remember: These deficiencies are intermediaries in amino acid catabolism. Here, propionyl-CoA is an intermediary in the oxidation of isoleucine, threonine, valine, and methionine.

In the early neonatal period, propionic acidemia can present as severe ketoacidosis with or without hyperammonemia. The infant will have encephalopathy, vomiting, and bone marrow depression. A late-onset complication is cardiomyopathy. Other infants may present with ketoacidosis precipitated by infection or vomiting.

Diagnose by examining urine organic acids. Look for large amounts of 3-hydroxypropionic and methylcitric acids. Abnormal ketone bodies are common too.

Treatment is dietary restriction of protein (usually < 1 g/kg/day) or the amino acids that are prone to produce more propionyl-CoA. Carnitine is helpful in increasing excretion of propionyl-CoA. Unfortunately, most die in early childhood. Other major problems include malnutrition with failure to thrive and recurrent infections; later, they can develop cardiomyopathy.

MULTIPLE CARBOXYLASE DEFICIENCY

This disorder is due to 1 of 2 defects in incorporating biotin into the carboxylases, acting on propionyl-CoA, 3-methylcrotonyl-CoA, acetyl-CoA, and pyruvate. The deficient enzymes are either holocarboxylase synthetase or biotinidase. Both deficiencies produce a triad: alopecia, skin rash, and encephalopathy. Seizures, hearing loss, and blindness can also be complications of untreated disease. Biotinidase deficiency usually presents later than holocarboxylase deficiency and has a periorificial dermatitis that looks like acrodermatitis enteropathica.

Diagnose by analyzing urine organic acid and finding increased 3-methylcrotonylglycine and 3-hydroxyisovaleric acid with lactic acids. Multiple carboxylase deficiency can also be found on newborn screening for biotinidase deficiency.

Treatment is quite effective with free biotin in doses of 5–20 mg/day. This will usually reverse all of the disease manifestations. Many states in the U.S. screen for biotinidase deficiency on newborn screening. Holocarboxylase deficiency should be detected with the expanded newborn panels.

METHYLMALONIC ACIDEMIAS

These are due to AR disorders that ultimately inhibit methylmalonyl-CoA mutase function. There are 4 different diseases that cause methylmalonic aciduria. These are mutase deficiency, cobalamin A deficiency, cobalamin B deficiency, and cobalamin C deficiency. Methylmalonic acidemias have many different forms, from defects in the mutase gene to a defect in the biosynthesis of adenosyl-B_{12} from vitamin B_{12}, its cofactor.

Clinically, these patients present early with hyperammonemia, ketoacidosis, and thrombocytopenia—or later with chronic ketotic hyperglycinemia, vomiting, and FTT. A late-onset complication is renal failure of uncertain origin, and cardiomyopathy can also occur.

Diagnose with organic acid analysis of urine, which will show increased methylmalonic acid and abnormal ketone bodies, as with propionic acidemia. Homocystinuria is also present if the patient has the enzyme deficit in the pathway that blocks the synthesis of methyl-B_{12}, resulting in increased methylmalonic acid and increased levels of homocysteine.

Treatment relies on restricting dietary protein. Carnitine is useful. Liver and kidney transplantation may be curative. If the patient has both methylmalonic aciduria and homocystinuria, treat with betaine (which provides another methyl donor for the conversion of homocysteine to methionine) and IM vitamin B_{12}. Again, these children, like all patients with metabolic disorders, need to be followed by a metabolic specialist and dietician.

DEFECTS IN FATTY ACID OXIDATION
OVERVIEW

Remember: Fatty acid oxidation occurs in the mitochondria, and this oxidation is what provides the main energy source for heart and skeletal muscle (see Figure 10-2). Also, fatty acid oxidation generates acetyl-CoA, which enters the Krebs cycle and thus provides energy to other tissues when the supply of glucose is gone. Fatty acids

initially are conjugated to carnitine. Then carnitine is transported across the mitochondrial membrane and released into the "matrix" as an acyl-CoA before it can be catabolized in the β-oxidation spiral.

Here is the rub: Diseases that limit β-oxidation do so by:
• reducing carnitine uptake by cells,
• inhibiting fatty acids themselves from entering mitochondria, or
• by blocking β-oxidation itself.

If β-oxidation is limited, there also is limited energy available for the heart and skeletal muscles at rest; it also limits the ability of the brain to cope with low-glucose settings; thus, it is the poster child for disorders of energy metabolism. These are more often AR disorders.

There are 12 known disorders affecting mitochondrial fatty acid oxidation and ketogenesis. Medium-chain acyl-CoA dehydrogenase (MCAD) deficiency is the most common. Age of onset varies from birth to adulthood. The most common clinical presentations involve the hepatic, skeletal, muscular, and cardiac systems. Neonates will present with arrhythmias (Makes sense, doesn't it? The heart cannot function correctly because of lack of energy.) and hypoglycemia. Sometimes, they will have facial dysmorphisms and renal cystic dysplasia. Older children will have arrhythmias or cardiomyopathies. Muscle weakness is common, as is exercise-induced rhabdomyolysis.

The main laboratory studies to detect these disorders:
• Routine lab measurements (CBC, electrolytes, liver function studies, ammonia, lactate, CPK)
• Free and acylcarnitine levels in the blood
• GC-MS analysis of organic acids
• Analysis of plasma acylcarnitine and urine acylglycines by specialized techniques

Definitive diagnosis of these disorders requires measurement of specific enzyme activity or mutation analysis.

Treat the acute presentation with IV 10% dextrose and possibly L-carnitine. Long-term therapy revolves around keeping the

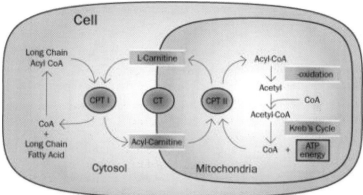

Figure 10-2: Fatty Acid Oxidation

notes

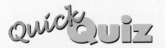
glucose from getting low, especially important when the patient is stressed by illness or decreased intake and catabolism.

We'll now discuss some of the more testable disorders.

CARNITINE UPTAKE DEFECT (1° CARNITINE DEFICIENCY)

This AR defect, located on chromosome 5, occurs in the plasma membrane of the cell. This disorder is caused by a deficiency of the carnitine transporter in the kidneys, where free carnitine is recycled for use by the body. When this transporter is not functioning, free carnitine is lost in the urine and results in low levels of free carnitine in serum. This defect responds very well to treatment with L-carnitine.

Patients will present in early infancy or later childhood with cardiomyopathy or recurrent episodes of encephalopathy and hypoketotic hypoglycemia. If the skeletal muscles are involved, weakness is prominent. Conduction defects and arrhythmias are rare with this disorder, in contrast to other disorders.

Diagnose by finding very low levels of carnitine in tissues. In serum, it may be undetectable or < 1 μmol/L. However, keep in mind that other losses from fatty acid oxygenation defects or organic acidurias can also cause fairly severe carnitine deficiency or secondary deficiency.

Treat with L-carnitine, which results in dramatic improvement. Administer orally for chronic maintenance, IV for emergencies.

DEFECTS OF FATTY ACID ENTRY INTO MITOCHONDRIA

Short- and medium-chain fatty acids can enter mitochondria directly, but CoA esters that are longer than 12 carbons require transport with carnitine palmitoyltransferases I and II (CPT I and CPT II) and by carnitine-acylcarnitine translocase. AR disorders occur and cause defects in these enzymes.

All of the transporter defects can present in infancy with fasting-induced hypoglycemia, liver failure, and cardiomyopathy. However, they all can have later phenotypes as well. You see the more common phenotype in adults, known as the "muscular" type. Here the patient has exercise-induced muscle pain and rhabdomyolysis.

The other phenotype of CPT II is very rare, occurs only in infants/children, and is a hepatocardiomuscular form. If it occurs early, the infants die in 1–2 weeks with complete liver and heart failure. Those presenting later with the rare phenotype of CPT II will have hypoketotic hypoglycemia, cardiomyopathy, and muscle disease.

Carnitine-acylcarnitine translocase deficiency presents in the newborn with hyperammonemia, conduction defects, and high CPK. Prognosis is good if the infant survives the early initial insult.

Diagnosis for CPT I: normal or elevated serum carnitine levels, and the serum-acylcarnitine profile is normal. In CPT II and translocase deficiency, serum-carnitine levels are very low with elevated C_{16} esters (an abnormal acylcarnitine profile).

Treat acute cases with IV glucose and aggressive hydration. Fasting prevention will alleviate symptoms. Give carnitine if serum-carnitine levels are low. Medium-chain triglycerides (MCT) oil, which can enter the mitochondria without these enzymes, provides an alternative energy source as well.

DEFECTS IN β-OXIDATION

Overview

Once acyl-CoA is in the mitochondria, it enters the β-oxidation cycle. Here, a series of reactions occurs, and defects/ deficiencies of the enzymes can cause problems. Different enzymes cleave different lengths of carbon chains.

3 main AR conditions will be discussed in this group:
1) Defects in very long-chain acyl-CoA dehydrogenase (VLCAD)
2) Defects in long-chain 3-hydroxyacyl-CoA dehydrogenase (LCHAD)
3) Defects in medium-chain acyl-CoA dehydrogenase (MCAD)

Very Long-chain Acyl-CoA Dehydrogenase (VLCAD) Deficiency

VLCAD presents in infancy as arrhythmias with severe cardiomyopathy and sudden death. You may occasionally see it in older infants and children with hepatic, cardiac, or muscular abnormalities. Diagnose by finding elevated saturated and unsaturated C_{14-18} esters. Free carnitine is usually low. The enzyme is located on chromosome 17. Treatment includes a high carbohydrate diet and avoiding fasting. If an acute episode occurs, give IV glucose and fluids. Frequent meals and avoiding fasting is the treatment of choice, especially for infants. You can use medium-chain triglycerides (MCT) because their oxidation does not involve VLCAD.

notes

Long-chain 3-hydroxyacyl-CoA Dehydrogenase (LCHAD) Deficiency

LCHAD is the long-chain-specific enzyme, and it acts on all acyl groups longer than 8 carbons. LCHAD deficiency can "stand alone" or be in conjunction with two other enzymes: long-chain enoyl-CoA hydratase and β-ketothiolase. Patients with the "stand alone" deficiency will usually present in infancy with fasting-induced hypoketotic hypoglycemia, although some will have cardiomyopathy or, later in adulthood, exercise-induced rhabdomyolysis. A clue in the history may be the pregnancy. Was it complicated with acute fatty liver or HELLP (hemolysis, elevated liver function tests, and low platelets) syndrome?

Patients with LCHAD deficiency frequently develop cholestatic liver disease and have retinopathy with hypopigmentation or focal pigment aggregations later in life. Note: These are not seen in MCAD or VLCAD deficiency!

Therapy is very similar to that for VLCAD and MCAD. Frequent meals, without prolonged fasting, are recommended, especially for infants. You also can use medium-chain triglycerides and carnitine. Oral docosahexaenoic acid may reverse retinopathy if it occurs.

Medium-chain Acyl-CoA Dehydrogenase (MCAD) Deficiency

MCAD deficiency usually presents in the first 2 years. The child will have fasting-induced lethargy and hypoglycemia. Seizures and coma are common. MCAD deficiency—as well as the majority of other fatty acid oxygenation disorders—has been implicated in some cases of Reye syndrome and SIDS. In an acute episode, you will usually see elevated liver transaminases and CPK with hypoglycemia. Liver biopsy will show microvesicular steatosis.

Diagnose MCAD deficiency by finding elevated C_8, $C_{8:1}$, and $C_{10:1}$ esters. Free-serum carnitine is low sometimes, but not consistently. The enzyme is on chromosome 1.

Acute treatment is IV glucose and bicarbonate. You cannot use medium-chain triglycerides because this acyl-CoA dehydrogenase is what is missing. This causes buildup of medium chains that in turn can be toxic to the cells.

Preventative maintenance includes avoiding fasting as appropriate for age when healthy. But during illness, rapid intervention is most important. Oral carnitine can be helpful if low, but this is controversial.

The majority of states screen newborns for MCAD deficiency because it responds so well to effective treatment. Prior to newborn screening, 25% of infants died with the first metabolic illness.

Glutaric Acidemia Type 2 (Multiple Acyl-CoA Dehydrogenase Deficiency)

This is due to defects in electron-transfer flavoprotein (ETF) and ETF:ubiquinone oxidoreductase (EFT:QO). These transfer electrons from acyl-CoA dehydrogenases involved in fatty acid and amino acid oxidation from FAD coenzymes into the respiratory chain. AR defects in these 2 enzymes cause glutaric acidemia Type 2.

The neonate may present with severe hypoglycemia, metabolic acidosis, hyperammonemia, and the odor of sweaty feet, as with isovaleric acidemia. Frequently, the patient has cardiomyopathy, facial dysmorphism, and severe renal cystic dysplasia.

Diagnose by finding glutarylcarnitine, isovalerylcarnitine, and straight-chain esters of 4, 8, 10, and 12 carbon-compound lengths. Serum carnitine is low and ketones are absent. Patients with absolute deficiency die in the first few weeks, usually due to conduction defects. Those with "incomplete" defects survive into adulthood.

Treatment relies on avoiding fasting and may require continuous intragastric feeds. Carnitine is useful. You cannot use medium-chain triglycerides because all of the acyl-CoA dehydrogenases are deficient.

DISORDERS OF CARBOHYDRATE METABOLISM (GLYCOGEN STORAGE DISEASES)

MONO- AND POLYSACCHARIDES

Essentially, 3 monosaccharides (glucose, fructose, and galactose) and 1 polysaccharide (glycogen) are relevant for disorders of the carbohydrate metabolism. Glucose is the main source of energy metabolism. When metabolized, glucose makes ATP via glycolysis (glucose is converted to pyruvate) or mitochondrial oxidative phosphorylation (pyruvate to carbon dioxide and water). Eating, gluconeogenesis, and breakdown of storage glycogen maintain glucose levels. Galactose is derived from lactose (galactose + glucose), which is in milk and milk products. Fructose is derived from sucrose (fructose + glucose) and fructose itself in the diet (fruits and vegetables). Glycogen is the storage form of glucose. Defects in glycogen metabolism usually lead to buildup of glycogen in tissues, resulting in glycogen storage diseases.

GLYCOGEN STORAGE DISEASES

Most of these diseases are inherited as AR traits (except for phosphoglycerate kinase deficiency and one form of phosphorylase kinase deficiency, which are both X-linked disorders). Frequency of all forms of glycogen storage diseases is about 1/20,000.

notes

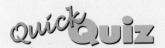

The most common disorders are:

- Glucose-6-phosphatase deficiency (Type I, von Gierke's)
- Lysosomal acid α-glucosidase deficiency (Type II, Pompe's)—does not present as an energy metabolic defect but is a lysosomal storage disease that has excess glycogen storage
- Debrancher deficiency (Type III)
- Liver phosphorylase kinase deficiency (Type IX)

The most common adult disorder is myophosphorylase deficiency (Type V, also known as McArdle disease). We will subdivide these glycogen storage diseases into those that more commonly affect the liver vs. those that more commonly affect muscle tissues.

CARBOHYDRATE METABOLISM DISORDERS PRESENTING AS HYPOGLYCEMIA AND HEPATOMEGALY

Type I Glycogen Storage Disease (Glucose-6-phosphatase/Translocase Deficiency, von Gierke Disease)

Type I glycogen storage disease is due to a defect in glucose-6-phosphatase in the liver, kidney, and intestinal mucosa. There are 2 subtypes: Ia: from a defective glucose-6-phosphatase enzyme; and Ib: from a defect in the translocase that transports glucose-6-phosphatase across the membrane. Both of these cause the same defect, which is failure to convert glucose-6-phosphatase to glucose in the liver. With this defect, the individual is likely to suffer from fasting hypoglycemia.

Clinically, these patients will present at about age 3–4 months with hepatomegaly, failure to thrive, and/or hypoglycemia with seizures—at a time when babies start to eat less often and parents are trying to have them sleep through the night. The kids have "doll-like faces with fat cheeks," thin extremities, short stature, and a large protuberant abdomen due to the hepatomegaly. The kidneys are also hypertrophied, but the spleen and heart are normal in size.

Things to look for specifically: hypoglycemia, lactic acidosis, hyperuricemia, and hyperlipidemia (increased VLDL, LDL, and apolipoproteins B, C, and E). Note: Even though these patients have hepatomegaly, the liver transaminases are usually normal. The plasma may appear "milky" because of the hypertriglyceridemia.

Types Ia and Ib are similar, except that Ib has associated, recurrent bacterial infections due to neutropenia and impaired neutrophil function. Oral and intestinal mucosa ulcers also occur with Type Ib.

In the long term, the liver is the most commonly affected organ, but other organ systems will also be affected. Gout will usually appear in puberty because of the elevated uric acid. Puberty itself is usually delayed but otherwise, sexual development is normal. Pancreatitis can occur because of the elevated lipids.

By age 20–30 years, most patients will develop hepatic adenomas that can bleed and occasionally become malignant. Pulmonary hypertension and osteoporosis can occur. Proteinuria occurs in all patients older than age 20. HTN, stones, and abnormal creatinine clearance are common. With advanced disease, focal segmental glomerulonephritis develops.

Diagnosis: You can usually suspect this disease clinically by finding abnormal lactate and lipid levels. Also, if you give glucagon or epinephrine, blood glucose levels will not rise, but lactate will. Gene-based mutation analysis will provide the definitive diagnosis. Liver biopsy is generally not required.

Aim treatment at preventing hypoglycemia with continuous nasogastric feeds or oral administration of uncooked cornstarch when the patient is old enough for pancreatic enzymes to break it down. Fructose and galactose cannot be converted to free glucose, so restrict these in the diet. Use allopurinol to lower uric acid levels. G-CSF has been used to correct the neutropenia of Ib-affected individuals. Some patients have difficulty with bleeding, especially during surgery, since they have platelet dysfunction. You can correct this with a constant infusion of glucose for 24–48 hours prior to surgery.

Type III Glycogen Storage Disease (Debrancher Deficiency, Limit Dextrinosis)

Type III is due to a deficiency of glycogen-debranching enzyme. This enzyme (along with phosphorylase) is responsible for complete degradation of glycogen. When the enzyme is deficient, a weird type of glycogen is formed that resembles limit dextrin. Type III is AR, occurs on chromosome 1, and has an increased incidence in non-Ashkenazi Jews of North African descent.

Patients with Type III present with:

- hepatomegaly,
- hypoglycemia,
- short stature,
- skeletal myopathy, and/or
- cardiomyopathy.

notes

In 85% of patients, it presents with both liver and muscle abnormalities; this is known as Type IIIa glycogen storage disease. In the other 15%, it involves only the liver and is known as Type IIIb glycogen storage disease.

It is difficult to clinically distinguish between Type III and Type I, but usually the kidneys are not enlarged in Type III. In Type III, the hepatomegaly and hepatic symptoms may improve after puberty, although some patients will go on to develop cirrhosis—particularly those of Japanese ancestry. Unlike Type I, the liver in Type III is fibrotic. Fasting ketosis is prominent in Type III, and, unlike Type I, lactate and uric acid are normal.

In Type IIIa, muscle weakness is minimal in children but becomes progressively worse by their 30s and 40s. In females, polycystic ovaries frequently occur, but infertility is not an issue.

In Type IIIa, deficient debranching enzyme activity can be demonstrated in the liver, skeletal muscle, and heart. In Type IIIb, only the liver is involved. DNA testing provides definitive diagnosis without need for liver or muscle biopsy in IIIb but is not available for IIIa.

Diet is less stringent in Type III than in Type I. Frequent high-carbohydrate meals are usually effective in preventing hypoglycemia. Also, patients do not need to restrict fructose and galactose, as do those with Type I.

With Type IIIb, liver symptoms usually improve with age and disappear after puberty. However, cirrhosis can occur later in life. In Type IIIa, muscle weakness/atrophy worsens in adulthood.

Type IV Glycogen Storage Disease
(Branching Enzyme Deficiency, Amylopectinosis, or Andersen Disease)

Deficiency of branching enzyme causes accumulation of an abnormal glycogen that has decreased solubility; its structure resembles amylopectin. It is a rare AR disorder and is located on chromosome 3.

There are many clinical presentations for this disorder but the most common is cirrhosis of the liver with hepatomegaly and FTT in the first 18 months of life. The cirrhosis is so severe that death usually occurs by age 5. The abnormal accumulation of the amylopectin-like material is widespread in the liver, heart, skin, brain, nerves, and intestine. There is also a neuromuscular form of this disorder.
Treatment is supportive, and there is no specific therapy.

Type VI Glycogen Storage Disease
(Liver Phosphorylase Deficiency—Hers Disease)

This is very rare, and it appears that patients with liver phosphorylase deficiency have a benign course. Those affected have hepatomegaly and growth retardation in childhood, but these resolve before or at puberty. No specific therapy is usually required.

Type IX Glycogen Storage Disease
(Liver Phosphorylase Kinase Deficiency)

Defects of phosphorylase kinase deficiency can cause various problems. 4 of them will be briefly discussed.
1) X-linked liver phosphorylase kinase deficiency: This is a very common liver glycogenosis. It typically presents within the first 5 years with hepatomegaly and growth retardation, but these conditions resolve by adulthood. Hypoglycemia is mild, if at all present. By adulthood, most individuals are completely asymptomatic, even though they have persistent deficiency. However, they may go on to develop cirrhosis and possibly require liver transplant.

2) Autosomal liver and muscle phosphorylase kinase deficiency: This is an AR form of phosphorylase kinase deficiency occurring in the liver and muscles. Its presentation is very similar to that of the X-linked form. Some will also have muscle hypotonia.

3) Autosomal liver phosphorylase kinase deficiency: This is the AR form of the X-linked disease mentioned above and involves only the liver. It is not benign like the X-linked form; many of these patients develop cirrhosis.

4) Muscle-specific phosphorylase kinase deficiency: This is the other X-linked disorder, and it causes cramps and myoglobinuria on exercise or progressive muscle weakness/atrophy. The enzyme is deficient only in muscle, not in the liver or in blood.

Type 0 Glycogen Storage Disease
(Glycogen Synthase Deficiency)

This is really not a glycogen storage disease, per se, because the enzyme deficiency leads to a decrease in glycogen stores. The enzyme is located on chromosome 12. Infants will present with early morning drowsiness and fatigue (hmm …) and sometimes seizures with hypoglycemia and hyper-ketonemia (okay, never mind). There is no hepatomegaly. Definitive diagnosis depends on liver biopsy to measure the enzyme activity. Treatment is symptomatic, involving frequent feedings rich in protein and a nighttime snack of uncooked cornstarch to prevent hypoglycemia. Most patients do well and survive into adulthood.

Type XI Glycogen Storage Disease
(Hepatic Glycogenesis with Renal Fanconi Syndrome; Known as Fanconi-Bickel Syndrome)

This is rare and occurs as an AR defect in the glucose transporter 2 (GLUT2) gene, which transports glucose in and out of the hepatic, pancreatic, intestinal, and renal epithelial cells. Patients have proximal renal tubular dysfunction and accumulation of glycogen in the liver and kidney. There are < 100 cases reported worldwide, but it does appear on Board exams. Look for parents who are consanguineous.

notes

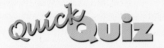

1) What causes Type IV glycogen storage disease?

2) How does a child with Type IV glycogen storage disease present?

3) What is different about Type 0 glycogen storage disease?

4) How does a child with Fanconi-Bickel syndrome present?

5) How does a child with Type V glycogen storage disease present?

6) What laboratory test is elevated at rest and after exercise in patients with McArdle disease?

7) What is the metabolic disorder in Pompe disease?

Children will present < 1 year of age with FTT, rickets, and a large, protuberant abdomen due to the hepatomegaly. Liver transaminases are normal, however. Oral galactose and glucose-tolerance tests show impaired tolerance. Diagnosis is by tissue biopsy; treatment is not very helpful, with growth retardation as the primary manifestation (e.g., poor height attainment).

CARBOHYDRATE METABOLISM DISORDERS THAT PRESENT WITH MUSCLE PROBLEMS

Overview

These disorders can be further separated, based on whether there also is cardiac involvement. Those without: Type V (McArdle disease) and Type VII (Tarui disease). Type II (Pompe disease) is the main one in the skeletal and/or cardiac category.

Type V Glycogen Storage Disease (Muscle Phosphorylase Deficiency or McArdle Disease)

Deficiency of this enzyme reduces ATP generation by glycogenolysis and results in glycogen accumulation. It is an AR disorder and is located on chromosome 11.

Symptoms are usually not present until patients reach their 20s and 30s, although many can remember symptoms from their childhood, including exercise-induced muscle cramps and exercise intolerance. The exercise can be either brief and intense, such as sprinting, or sustained, less intense activity, such as walking up a hill. Many patients report a "second-wind" phenomenon. If they rest, they can resume the exercise. 50% will report burgundy-colored urine after exercise, which is from myoglobinuria due to rhabdomyolysis.

CPK is elevated at rest and increases after exercise. Exercise will also increase ammonia and uric acid in the blood.

What suggests the diagnosis? Exercising the patient and not finding an increase in blood lactate level, but instead finding an increased ammonia level. This suggests a defect in the conversion of glycogen or glucose to lactate. Enzymatic assays on muscle tissue or DNA analysis for the myophosphorylase gene will provide definitive diagnosis.

Gear treatment toward avoidance of strenuous exercise since you want to prevent rhabdomyolysis from occurring. Gradual aerobic training or oral fructose/glucose intake can improve exercise tolerance.

Type VII Glycogen Storage Disease (Muscle Phosphofructokinase Deficiency or Tarui Disease)

This deficiency is due to a lack of muscle phosphofructokinase, which causes fructose-6-phosphate to become fructose-1, 6-diphosphate. It is an AR disorder, very rare, and mainly reported in people of Japanese descent or Ashkenazi Jews.

The symptoms are similar to Type V—early onset of fatigue and pain with exercise.

However, Type VII differs from Type V in the following ways:
1) It is usually present in childhood.
2) Hemolysis occurs.
3) Increased uric acid levels are common.
4) An amylopectin-like glycogen is deposited in muscle fibers.
5) Exercise intolerance is much worse after a carbohydrate-loaded meal; glucose can't be used by the muscle, and the presence of the glucose inhibits the ability of the lipolysis to provide the muscle with energy via fatty acids and ketones.

Remember: With Type V, glucose consumption before exercise helps.

Diagnosis: Find the defect in affected tissues through biochemical or histochemical means. Aim treatment toward preventing strenuous exercise.

Type II Glycogen Storage Disease (Acid α-1,4-glucosidase Deficiency or Pompe Disease)

This does not fall into an energy metabolism defect category; it is a lysosomal storage defect with excess storage of glycogen.

This disease is due to a deficiency in the lysosomal acid α-1,4-glucosidase (also known as acid maltase), which is responsible for breaking down glycogen in lysosomal vacuoles. This disease is different in that the glycogen accumulates in the lysosomes, as opposed to accumulating in the cytoplasm as it does in the other glycogen storage diseases. It is an AR disorder on chromosome 17. Symptoms are from buildup of complex molecules, not primarily from energy problems.

Pompe disease has a wide variety of phenotypic presentations.
1) Infantile-onset form: This is the most severe and presents with cardiomegaly, hypotonia, and death before 1 year of age. The infant is normal at birth but soon develops generalized muscle weakness, macroglossia, hepatomegaly, and CHF due to hypertrophic cardiomyopathy. ECG shows a high-voltage QRS and a shortened PR interval.
2) Juvenile/late childhood form: Slowly progressive skeletomuscular manifestations without cardiac involvement. Patients may present with slowed developmental milestones, such as delayed walking. Swallowing difficulties, proximal muscle weakness, and respiratory muscle depression then follow. Death may occur before these individuals reach their 20s.
3) Adult form: This presents in those 20–70 years of age as a slowly progressive myopathy without cardiac involvement. Clinically, patients have progressive proximal muscle weakness, including the trunk. Lower extremities are more severely affected than the upper extremities. The pelvic girdle and diaphragm are most seriously affected. Initially, the adult might present with increased sleepiness, morning headache, and exertional dyspnea.

Look for elevated CPK, AST, and LDH, especially in the infantile form. Muscle biopsy will show vacuoles that are full of glycogen on staining.

Diagnosis: Find reduced or absent levels of acid-glucosidase activity in muscle or skin fibroblasts. Enzyme-replacement therapy is now available. In the juvenile and adult forms, institute a high-protein diet. Nocturnal ventilatory support may be necessary and will improve daytime symptoms.

GALACTOSE METABOLISM DISORDERS

These fall into the intoxification classification. The symptoms are secondary to buildup of toxic metabolites.

Galactose 1-phosphate Uridyl Transferase Deficiency or Galactosemia

[Know this!] Galactosemia will be on your Board exam at least 2 or 3 times. It occurs in 1/60,000 births and is inherited as an AR disorder. There are several enzymatic variations in the population. The Duarte variant is the most common form, and has a carrier frequency of 12% in the population! Those with Duarte-variant homozygote have about 50% of normal red cell enzyme activity, but do not have symptoms. Those with Duarte galactosemia (D/G) compound heterozygosity have only 25% activity, with elevated galactose 1-phosphate levels. Again, these patients are usually asymptomatic, but most practitioners would restrict lactose intake if the RBC galactose 1-phosphate levels are elevated.

What happens? The normal infant receives 20% of its caloric intake as lactose, which, as you remember, consists of glucose and galactose. With deficiency of galactose 1-phosphate uridyltransferase, the infant cannot metabolize galactose 1-phosphate, and this accumulates in the kidney, liver, and brain.

Clinically, with classic galactosemia these infants have some combination of:
- Jaundice
- Hepatosplenomegaly
- Hypoglycemia
- Irritability
- Cataracts
- Cirrhosis
- Mental retardation
- Vomiting
- Seizures
- Lethargy
- Poor weight gain
- Vitreous hemorrhage
- Ascites

Those affected are at increased risk for *E. coli* sepsis, which usually precedes the diagnosis of galactosemia.

Suspect this disorder when you discover a reducing substance in urine while the patient is drinking breast milk, cow's milk, or formula containing lactose; but this is neither sensitive nor specific to confirm or rule out the diagnosis. Definitive diagnosis requires deficient activity of galactose 1-phosphate uridyltransferase (GALT) in RBCs or other tissues, while also showing an increased concentration of galactose 1-phosphatase.

Newborn screening for galactosemia is widespread; use a fluorescent spot test (Beutler test) for GALT activity for diagnosis of galactosemia.

Elimination of galactose from the diet reverses growth failure and renal/hepatic problems. Even the cataracts will regress. Prognosis is improved, but long-term effects are still common: ovarian failure, amenorrhea, developmental delay, and learning disabilities that increase with age. Speech disorders are also very common. We know that control of galactose 1-phosphate levels alone does not correlate with outcome, so other "yet to be determined" factors must be involved.

Galactokinase Deficiency

Cataracts alone typically manifest this disorder. Otherwise, the infant is asymptomatic. The defect is found on chromosome 17. Treatment is dietary restriction of galactose.

Uridine-diphosphate Galactose 4-epimerase (UDP Gal 4-epimerase) Deficiency

The accumulated metabolites are very similar to those seen in galactosemia; but there is also an increase in cellular UDP-galactose. This deficiency may not be detected on a newborn screen.

There are two forms of this disease:
1) Benign form: Individuals are healthy and no treatment is necessary. The only evidence is seen in red blood cells.
2) Generalized form: Clinically resembles galactosemia, with the additional symptoms of hypotonia and nerve deafness. Treatment with dietary restriction of galactose is effective.

notes

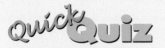

The galactose 1-phosphate uridyltransferase activity is normal, unlike in classic galactosemia.

FRUCTOSE METABOLISM DISORDERS

These fall into the intoxification classification. The symptoms are secondary to buildup of toxic metabolites.

Benign Fructosuria (Deficiency of Fructokinase)

This is benign, requires no treatment, and has no clinical manifestations. It is an incidental finding when you discover fructose during urine screen for reducing substances.

Deficiency of Fructose 1,6-bisphosphate Aldolase (Aldolase B, or Hereditary Fructose Intolerance)

This is a severe disease of infancy and appears when the infant ingests fructose-containing food. The deficient enzyme causes the hydrolysis of fructose 1-phosphate and fructose 1,6-biphosphate into 3 sugars: dihydroxyacetone phosphate, glyceraldehyde 3-phosphate, and glyceraldehyde. Deficiency of the enzyme causes an accumulation of fructose 1-phosphate and leads to severe toxic symptoms when exposed to fructose.

Most believe this disorder to be fairly common at 1/23,000; the gene is isolated on chromosome 9. Point mutations are common in Europe and the United States, with proline replacing an alanine.

Those affected are completely healthy until they ingest fructose or sucrose (table sugar). Usually, the culprit is juice or sweetened cereal. It can look a lot like galactosemia but onset is generally later, when exposed to the sugars as opposed to the first week or so of life: jaundice, hepatomegaly, vomiting, lethargy, seizures, and irritability. Laboratory results will show prolonged clotting time, low albumin, elevated bilirubin and transaminases, and proximal tubular dysfunction. If the sugar intake is continued, severe hypoglycemia occurs, followed by liver and kidney failure, and death.

Suspect this deficiency if you find fructose as a urinary-reducing substance during an episode. Also, you can do an IV fructose tolerance test. Giving the IV fructose will result in a rapid drop in serum phosphate and glucose before a subsequent rise in magnesium and uric acid, so be very careful in monitoring during the test. (Note: Do not use oral fructose!)

A definitive diagnosis depends on assaying fructose 1,6-biphosphate aldolase B activity in the liver.

Treatment consists of completely ridding the diet of all sources of sucrose, fructose, and sorbitol. Treatment will reverse the liver and kidney damage, as well as spur growth. Mental retardation is very uncommon. Most symptoms improve with age.

GLUCONEOGENESIS DISORDERS

Fructose 1,6-diphosphatase Deficiency

This is a defect in gluconeogenesis found on chromosome 9. Patients will have severe episodes of metabolic acidosis, hypoglycemia, hyperventilation, seizures, and coma. Decrease in oral intake during an illness or gastroenteritis initiates events. This contrasts with hereditary fructose intolerance, where renal and liver functions are normal. Treat with IV glucose. For the long term, patients must avoid fasting and eliminate fructose/sucrose from the diet. Cornstarch is helpful for preventing hypoglycemia. Diagnose by finding the enzyme deficiency in liver or intestinal biopsy.

Phosphoenolpyruvate Carboxylase (PEPCK) Deficiency

PEPCK is key in gluconeogenesis. It causes oxaloacetate to become phosphoenolpyruvate. It is very rare.

OXIDATIVE PHOSPHORYLATION DISEASES AND DISORDERS OF PYRUVATE OXIDATION

MITOCHONDRIAL DNA MUTATIONS

Overview

All disorders of mitochondrial DNA (mtDNA) are maternally inherited, but not all mitochondrial disorders are caused by mtDNA mutations—the majority have autosomal recessive inheritance, but they could also be autosomal dominant or X-linked. By definition, these are energy metabolism defects.

The diseases below are based on phenotype. Not all have the same genetic mutations and the mutations found can vary in the family.

notes

Kearns-Sayre and Chronic, Progressive External Ophthalmoplegia (CPEO) Syndromes

The following triad classifies these syndromes: ptosis, ophthalmoplegia, and ragged-red fiber myopathy. This triad is very specific for the presence of a mitochondrial DNA (mtDNA) mutation.

Kearns-Sayre syndrome is the most severe and can begin in infancy, childhood, or adolescence. In addition to the triad, multisystem disease is common, particularly including:

• cardiomyopathies,
• diabetes mellitus,
• cerebellar ataxia, and
• deafness.

Some may present in infancy with a variant called Pearson syndrome, which has pancytopenia and pancreatitis (think Ps).

CPEO-plus is a disorder of intermediate severity that begins in adolescence or adulthood and has variable systemic involvement, including the eyelids and eye muscles.

Isolated CPEO is the mildest variant, but clinical signs/symptoms worsen with age. These individuals can progress to CPEO-plus or Kearns-Sayre syndrome.

These 3 variants are usually due to a rearrangement of mtDNA. Most of the mutations are spontaneous events during oogenesis or early embryogenesis and not inherited. They can also occur as nuclear DNA mutations and be transmitted in an autosomal dominant or recessive fashion.

Myoclonic Epilepsy and Ragged-red Fiber Disease (MERRF)

MERRF usually begins anytime from late childhood to adulthood. The 3 common things you see in this disorder are:

1) Epilepsy
2) Cerebellar ataxia
3) Ragged-red fiber myopathy

Myoclonic jerks occur at rest and increase in frequency/amplitude with movement. Most of these are due to an A-to-G mutation of a nucleotide in tRNA of mitochondrial DNA.

Mitochondrial Encephalomyopathy, Lactic Acidosis, and Stroke-like Episodes (MELAS)

MELAS can appear at any age, but mostly present before 45 years of age, and are known as "stroke of the young." The stroke can be associated with migraines, seizures, or both. It can be difficult to distinguish MELAS from other causes of stroke, especially now that we are seeing more young people with atherosclerotic disease. Look for myopathy, ataxia, cardiomyopathy, and diabetes mellitus presenting before the stroke. You will most commonly see cerebellar ataxia well before the stroke. The gene mutation is an A-to-G mutation in tRNA and is maternally inherited. Note: As many as 1% of patients with adult-onset diabetes mellitus may have the mutation, which brings an increased risk of stroke. Think of an oxidative phosphorylation disease in any young person with diabetes mellitus and stroke.

Leigh Syndrome

Consider Leigh syndrome (also known as subacute necrotizing encephalopathy) when you see cranial nerve findings, respiratory dysfunction, and ataxia with bilateral hyperintense signals on T_2-weighted MRI of the basal ganglia, cerebellum, or brainstem. It usually occurs during infancy/early childhood. Mitochondrial DNA mutations are usually responsible, although it can occur as nuclear DNA mutations, and it is transmitted as AR. Besides the findings listed above, patients can have cardiomyopathy, sensory and motor neuropathies, and muscle weakness.

Mitochondrial DNA Depletion Disorders

These disorders present in neonates and infants with:

• mitochondrial myopathy,
• hypotonia,
• liver dysfunction,
• progressive external ophthalmoplegia, and
• severe lactic acidosis.

There is a quantitative reduction in the number of mtDNA. Diagnose by Southern blot analysis, which will show that the copy number of mitochondrial DNA is greatly reduced in affected tissues.

Friedrich Ataxia

Technically, this is not a mitochondrial disorder, but it is transmitted as an AR disorder and mapped to chromosome 9. It occurs in about 1/50,000.

Symptoms of Friedrich ataxia include:

• Hypoactive or absent deep tendon reflexes
• Ataxia
• Corticospinal tract dysfunction
• Impaired vibratory and proprioceptive function
• Hypertrophic cardiomyopathy
• Diabetes mellitus

MUCOPOLYSACCHARIDOSES, MUCOLIPIDOSES, AND GLYCOPROTEINOSES

All symptoms result from lysosomal storage of large complex molecules; thus, these are complex molecule defects. (Remember: This is where Pompe disease fits in but it was initially classified as a glycogen storage disease.)

notes

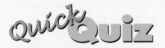

MUCOPOLYSACCHARIDOSES (MPS)

Overview

This group of disorders is a result of a defect in the catabolism of glycosaminoglycans. Depending on the disorder, you see accumulation of dermatan sulfate, heparan sulfate, or keratan sulfate. Lysosomes are cytoplasmic organelles that have enzymes with phagocytosis (degradation) of the micro-molecules (mucopolysaccharides, glycoproteins, and various lipids). These disorders result in accumulation of macro-molecules in target organs. Various lysosomal hydrolase enzymes are the culprits.

Infants are normal at birth, and the phenotypic characteristics of the disease appear over time as storage material accumulates. Exceptions are mucolipidosis Type II (I-cell disease) and G_{M1}-gangliosidosis, which will present in infancy. All disorders are progressive, and most are fatal. Most of these are more commonly known by their mnemonic name (MPS 1H = Hurler's, etc.).

Presentation is usually 1 of 3 forms:
- Dysmorphic/coarse features syndrome: MPS 1H, MPS II, MPS VI
- Learning difficulties, behavior problems, and dementia: MPS III
- Severe bone dysplasia: MPS IV

Screen urine first, but inaccurate/false-negative results are common. WBC and plasma lysosomal enzyme studies can be helpful. Also diagnostic are radiographs to look for dysostosis multiplex. Several of these disorders have enzyme-replacement therapy available commercially and newer drugs are undergoing clinical trials.

Mucopolysaccharidosis Type I (Hurler Syndrome)

MPS Type I is due to a defect in the gene coding for α-L-iduronidase on chromosome 4p16.3. There are wide variations in disease presentations. Those severely affected are frequently diagnosed within the first 2 years of life. They have coarsened facial features, with mid-face hypoplasia and large tongues. Early on, they will have frequent URIs and may have inguinal/umbilical hernias. Head circumference is usually > the 95th percentile, and communicating hydro-cephalus is common. Obstructive sleep apnea is also common, and ENT specialists are usually necessary for surgical help. Skeletal growth is usually normal during the first year, but severe growth retardation soon develops. These kids are at high risk for atlantoaxial subluxation. Systemically, you will find hepatosplenomegaly and cardiac disease. Corneal clouding and deafness are common. Prognosis is generally related to the cardiac involvement, which can be severe— with early cardiomyopathy and death. Older children frequently have mitral and atrial valvular involvement. Early coronary artery disease is common.

You may not see those less severely affected until early adulthood. Usually, they will present with bone abnormalities (spondylolisthesis of L5/S1, degenerative bone loss) or eye problems (corneal clouding and retinal disease). There is a variant called MPS IS (Scheie syndrome), in which patients have normal intelligence and life span; carpal tunnel syndrome is characteristic in this form.

Hematopoietic stem cell transplant (HSCT) has been successful in children < 18 months of age to prevent intellectual deterioration and has now been shown to provide a good chance for long-term survival. However, complex spinal surgery is still required because the HSCT does not correct the skeletal abnormalities. It appears that HSCT is useful only for MPS Types I and VI (VI is very rare and not discussed here). Treatment of choice is enzyme-replacement therapy for those with milder forms and later onset of symptoms.

Mucopolysaccharidosis Type II (Hunter Syndrome)

MPS II is due to a defect in the gene that encodes for iduronate-2-sulfatase on chromosome Xq27-28. Therefore, you will see it only in males (except for the rare female patient who has a chromosomal translocation or nonrandom X-inactivation). Clinically, these patients can present with a very wide range of findings. If children are severely affected, it can look like MPS I, but milder, because most live into their mid-teens. In milder forms of MPS II, normal life span is possible, as is the ability to reproduce and have normal intelligence. Two things to know about MPS II, as compared with MPS I: MPS II is inherited as X-linked recessive (the only one that is X-linked), and corneal clouding does not occur.

In those severely affected, diagnosis is usually made by 2 years of age.

Common findings are:
- learning difficulties (with challenging behavior, ADD, or seizures),
- middle ear disease,
- hernias,
- coarse facial appearance,
- diarrhea,
- joint stiffness, and
- hepatosplenomegaly.

A nodular rash around the scapulae and the extensor surfaces is pathognomonic (but rare in children). Cardiomyopathy is rare, but uncomplicated valvular lesions are relatively common.

notes

Atlantoaxial instability, as seen in MPS I, is not common in MPS II. However, you may see cervical cord compression leading to cervical myelopathy. Adults with MPS II have upper respiratory obstruction and sleep apnea.

Enzyme-replacement therapy is now available clinically. However, it has not proven to be useful in reversing skeletal symptoms, and CNS involvement does not seem to be affected.

Mucopolysaccharidosis Type III (Sanfilippo Syndrome)

There are 4 described variants of MPS III. Type A and B MPS III genes have been located on chromosome 17, resulting in an inability to catabolize heparan sulfate. The other 2 forms, C and D, are rarer and found on other chromosomes. The disease is usually diagnosed ~ age 4–5 years, with severe CNS involvement and mild somatic disease. This disproportionate involvement of the CNS is unique among the mucopolysaccharidoses. It usually follows a classic triphasic pattern: Several different genetic causes with similar phenotypes distinguished by different enzyme defects.

• Phase 1: Developmental delay alone with recurrent URIs, diarrhea, and sleep disturbance occurring before 1 year of age.
• Phase 2: Severe, challenging behavior with hyperactivity and aggression. These children have no conception of danger to themselves and must be watched continuously. Family life is completely uprooted. Major tranquilizers are usually required to sedate the child and modify the aggressive behavior. Precocious puberty is common, as well as progressive loss of motor skills.
• Phase 3: Swallowing dysfunction develops with further deterioration to a vegetative state by the mid-teens. Death occurs by the 20s.

Mucopolysaccharidosis Type IV (Morquio Syndrome)

MPS IV is due to a deficiency of galactose-6-sulfatase, resulting in defective degradation of keratan sulfate. MPS IV characteristics include short-trunk dwarfism, fine corneal deposits, and skeletal (spondyloepiphyseal) dysplasia distinct from other types of MPS, along with normal intelligence. The defect is on chromosome 16.

These patients present during the first year of life with severe skeletal dysplasia, but are not dysmorphic. Vertebral platyspondylisis is common.

Adults with the severe form are < 3½ feet in height and have:
• Fixed hip flexion
• Genu valgum
• Pes planus
• Sternal protrusion
• Short neck

Odontoid dysplasia is a universal, and the most severe, manifestation and results in progressive cervical myelopathy.

Most of the bone deformities cannot be corrected, and most patients eventually require motorized wheelchairs. Dental decay is also common.

MUCOLIPIDOSES (ML)

Mucolipidosis Type I (Cherry-red Spot Myoclonus Syndrome)

ML I has a wide range of presentations—from hydrops fetalis in infancy to juvenile sialidosis, myoclonus/ataxia, and a macular cherry-red spot. Most commonly, it presents between these two extremes with a mild Hurler-like phenotype and a cherry-red spot. Death occurs in the late teens.

Mucolipidosis Type II (I-cell Deficiency)

ML II presents as a defect in the post-translational modification of lysosomal enzymes, where a target sequence (mannose-6-phosphate) fails to attach to the enzyme. This causes the lysosomal enzymes to be "lost" in the extracellular spaces, because they can't be directed to the lysosomes. Without the lysosomal enzymes, the lysosomes can't break down a variety of substrates. As the substrates accumulate in the lysosome, they become toxic to the cell and inhibit cellular function. ML II causes severe clinical and radiologic abnormalities—and looks like Hurler syndrome in terms of physical findings. Periosteal, new bone formation is prominent. Hyperplastic gums are the clue to look for (so, a Hurler syndrome with hyperplastic gums). Unlike with the other disorders in this group, the head circumference is usually small. Death occurs early due to infection or cardiac failure.

Mucolipidosis Type III (Pseudo-Hurler Polydystrophy)

This is usually a milder disorder with later onset of clinical symptoms, between ages 2 and 4 years, with survival into the 60s. Approximately 50% of patients will have some learning disabilities or mental retardation. The main problem is orthopedic, with severe joint stiffness. Patients cannot raise their arms above their heads and also have progressive hip dysplasia. Carpal tunnel syndrome and cardiac valvular lesions are common. Patients share many features with MPS I and VI, but have no mucopolysacchariduria.

GLYCOPROTEINOSES

Note

There are numerous rare disorders due to these deficiencies. Only the most common or most tested are listed here.

Mannosidosis

This is usually due to α-mannosidase deficiency. It can present as Hurler-like early in infancy or as a more chronic form later in life. Immunologic abnormalities are most common, and upper respiratory infections prevail.

notes

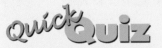
Others

Salla diseases—sialic-acid-transporter defect and infantile sialic-acid-storage disease—are very rare and mainly seen in those of Finnish descent. The infantile form is severe, and these infants present with hydrops fetalis, severe infections, and FTT. Salla disease is less severe and presents mainly with learning difficulties.

SPHINGOLIPIDOSES
OVERVIEW

Sphingolipidoses are characterized by defects in the lysosomal breakdown of sphingolipids. Again, these are disorders of complex molecules. When the deficient enzymes can't break down the lipids effectively, you get a buildup of ceramide, which is the lipophilic core. You also get a buildup of one of 2 hydrophilic compounds: either oligosaccharide (comprising the glycosphingolipids) or phosphorylcholine (which is sphingomyelin). Now the glycosphingolipids can be divided into 3 groups:
1) Globosides (red cell membranes and kidney)
2) Gangliosides (gray matter of the brain in synaptic terminals)
3) Galactocerebrosides (cerebral white matter)

Thus, if you know which "side" is involved, you can figure out where the problem will occur! The glycosphingolipids (globosides, gangliosides, and galactocerebrosides) and sphingomyelin are mainly components of cell membranes.

We'll now run through these disorders, based on age of presentation at onset, from neonatal through adulthood.

NEONATAL

Neonatal Gaucher Disease (Type 4)

These infants present with severe Gaucher disease and have thick, shiny, collodion skin. They have multiple congenital anomalies, hepatosplenomegaly, hypertonic and hyperreflexic movements, neck retraction, and a poor sucking mechanism. Nonimmune hydrops can be severe. They usually die within days or weeks.

1–6 MONTHS OF AGE

Gaucher Disease, Type 2 (Acute Neuronopathy)

This is rare and is due to a deficiency of lysosomal glucocerebrosidase. It involves increased accumulation of glucocerebroside in the brain and reticuloendothelial system. Infants are usually normal initially; but by age 2–4 months, they start having feeding difficulties and FTT. They develop strabismus, difficulty swallowing, and opisthotonic posturing. They have huge livers and spleens, but their liver function tests are usually only mildly affected. In a few infants, you can see a macular cherry-red spot.

A characteristic lab result to look for is an increased plasma tartrate-resistant acid phosphatase. Bone marrow aspiration shows classic Gaucher-storage cells—large, mononucleated histiocytes with cytoplasm containing basophilic material that looks like wrinkled tissue paper. Unlike the later presenting forms of Gaucher disease, skeletal involvement is minimal.

You can confirm diagnosis by finding a deficiency of β-glucosidase in the leukocytes or cultured fibroblasts. Treatment for Type 2 is supportive. Bone marrow transplant is not helpful. Most of these infants die before 2 years of age due to FTT or pneumonia.

Niemann-Pick Disease, Type A

This is a very rare form of Niemann-Pick disease (see below). It is a degenerative, neurovisceral disease occurring mainly in Ashkenazi Jews and is a deficiency of acid sphingomyelinase occurring on chromosome 11. It initially causes vomiting, diarrhea, and FTT. Hepatosplenomegaly is prominent. Neurologic problems occur ~ 5–10 months of age with hypotonia, progressive loss of motor skills, and reduction in spontaneous movements. 50% of those affected will have macular cherry-red spots, but usually these don't appear until after the occurrence of advanced neurologic disease.

Diagnose by finding low levels of sphingomyelinase in leukocytes or cultured fibroblasts.

6 MONTHS–2 YEARS

Gaucher Disease, Type 3 (Subacute Neuronopathy)

This is, again, due to deficiency of lysosomal glucocerebrosidase. Previously, most thought of it as uncommon, and that it occurred only in those of Swedish descent. Now we know it crosses all ethnic groups. There are 2 main groups for presentation: 3a and 3b. 3a has more prominent neurologic findings with little visceral involvement; 3b has prominent, severe visceral involvement.

3a will present in early-middle childhood with myoclonus, dementia, and ataxia. Look for isolated, horizontal supranuclear gaze palsy. You'll see blinking and superimposed upward looping of the eyes, and head thrusting. Tonic-clonic seizures are common later, along with spasticity.

notes

Hepatosplenomegaly is common, but not as severe as in 3b. Patients generally die before 30 years of age.

3b cases appear as though they have severe Type 1 at ~ age 2–3 years (see next page). The degree of hepatosplenomegaly is impressive and rapidly progressive compared to Type 1. Hepatocellular dysfunction is prominent with FTT, ascites, nosebleeds, and easy bruising. Portal hypertension and esophageal varices are common. The progression in the viscera is so rapid that neurologic manifestations are usually masked or never develop. The main finding of neurologic significance may be oculomotor apraxia: eye movements are not well executed.

Bone marrow will show the Gaucher cells. Confirm diagnosis by looking for deficiency of β-glucosidase in leukocytes or cultured skin fibroblasts. Bone marrow transplant is very effective in reversing the visceral and hematologic problems. We don't know the impact yet of bone marrow transplant on neurologic deterioration.

Niemann-Pick Disease, Type C

This is very common (well, common for these diseases anyway) and occurs in 250–500 children (1/150,000) each year in the U.S. The defect is not a lysosomal enzyme disorder, but instead it is likely due to routing of cholesterol esters within and through the lysosome. Cholesterol accumulates within the lysosomes of the reticuloendothelial system. It is put with the lysosomal deficiency disorders because it was classified before we had the molecular genetic know-how to classify it correctly; but it does appear to cause secondary buildup of GM2-gangliosidosis. Most cases have been mapped to chromosome 18.

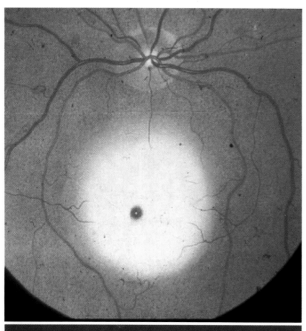

Figure 10-3: Tay-Sachs Cherry-red Spot

Most cases occur in ages 3–5 years, with signs of ataxia and hepatosplenomegaly. In older children, the 6–12-year range, presentation will usually include poor school performance and impaired fine motor skills. Organomegaly generally occurs but may not be present in up to 10% of cases. Cataplexy (e.g., sudden loss of motor movement after an emotional scare) and narcolepsy (uncontrolled attacks of sleep during the day) are common. On physical examination, the most common finding is supranuclear, vertical-gaze palsy (downward, upward, or both). Voluntary, vertical eye movement is lost, but reflex "doll's eye" movements are preserved. Dysphagia is common and may result in the need for a feeding tube. Death in the teenage years is common.

Another possible phenotype is isolated organomegaly. This is being further examined and is likely underdiagnosed.

Diagnosis: Demonstrate intralysosomal accumulation of unesterified cholesterol in cultured fibroblasts.

Tay-Sachs Disease

There are two forms: 1) infantile and 2) juvenile/adult.

1) The infantile form usually begins within the first few months of life and is due to β-hexosaminidase α-subunit deficiency. The first symptom is frequently an enhanced startle reflex to noise or light and quick extension of the arms and legs with clonic movements. Unlike the Moro reflex, this does not diminish with repeated stimuli. Motor skills are progressively lost. Axial hypotonia, extremity hypertonia, and hyperreflexia are common. In > 90% of infants, a macular cherry-red spot occurs. (See Figure 10-3.) This is due to storage of lipids (causes white discoloration) everywhere in the retina except the fovea, which remains the normal red color of the retina. Macrocephaly is common. Auditory stimuli cause seizures. Visceral organs are normal. By age 2–3 years, the child is decerebrate, blind, and unable to respond to stimuli. Autonomic dysfunction also occurs. By age 4–5 years, the child frequently has pneumonia.

2) The juvenile/adult form occurs in Ashkenazi Jews, with an indolent presentation. Early in childhood, the children are labeled "clumsy and awkward." The first sign may be an intention tremor (usually within the first 10 years). School problems may occur early on with dysarthria. By adolescence, proximal muscle weakness occurs with fasciculations and atrophy. Psychiatric symptoms are common and include anxiety, depression, and suicide. Usually, they can continue to ambulate until their 60s with appropriate help.

2–18 YEARS

Gaucher Disease, Type 1

Gaucher disease, Type 1 (3 types) is the most common lysosomal storage disease and is due to a deficiency of lysosomal glucocerebrosidase. It causes disease in 1/900

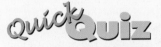
Ashkenazi Jews and has a carrier rate in this group of 1/15. This is a non-CNS disease with only visceral involvement. Splenomegaly is the most common presentation, and you will usually find it incidentally on a routine physical examination. Abdominal protuberance is common. The hypersplenism predisposes to significant thrombocytopenia, which can result in severe bleeding. Younger children may complain of "growing pains" in the lower extremities, especially at night, and there may be bone infiltration of storage cells. Growth retardation is common in those with severe disease.

At examination, look for a pale, anemic-like complexion associated with increased pigmentation of the skin. Generally, though, these children look well considering the extent of splenomegaly they have.

Bone marrow studies will show Gaucher storage cells. Confirm diagnosis by finding a deficiency of β-glucosidase in leukocytes or cultured skin fibroblasts.

The best treatment is enzyme-replacement therapy. Splenectomy is contraindicated because it causes increased storage in the lysosomes in the bone, resulting in worse bone disease. Bone crises usually require narcotics. Enzyme-replacement therapy is standard, with biweekly infusions of glucocerebrosidase. This reverses the hematologic and early skeletal complications of the disease. Note: Enzyme therapy does not work for the neurologic disease of Types 2 and 3!

Points to remember about the types of Gaucher disease:

Type 1: The most common and does not have CNS involvement.

Type 3: Neurologic symptoms are later in onset and more chronic than Type 2.

All forms: Hepatosplenomegaly, bone lesions, and some lung disease.

Diagnosis: 97% of mutations in Ashkenazi Jews, as compared to ~ 75% in the non-Jewish population, can be detected by screening for the 5 most common mutations.

Niemann-Pick Disease, Type B

Niemann-Pick disease, Type B, is due to incomplete deficiency of acid sphingomyelinase, and also is most common in Ashkenazi Jews. It is the same disease as Type A Niemann-Pick but has more residual enzyme activity. Clinically, it looks and presents just like Type 1 Gaucher disease, with isolated splenomegaly. Bone marrow studies will show the foamy storage histocytes, as seen in Niemann-Pick disease, Type A; but in Type B, the marrow also contains sea-blue histiocytes. Treatment is supportive, but severe disease appears to respond to bone marrow transplant.

Fabry Disease

Fabry disease is the only sphingolipidosis transmitted as an X-linked recessive disease; thus, it mainly affects boys. However, some heterozygous girls will develop similar pain crises. Boys present at puberty with complaints of severe, episodic pain in the hands and feet. Fever and increased ESR are common with the pain crises. Heat exposure, especially during physical exertion, will set off the pain crises, and the patient will not sweat, or will sweat very little (hypohidrosis). Usually, by the mid-to-late teenage years, the affected boys will develop angiokeratomata—tiny, red-to-dark blue, papular lesions on the buttocks, scrotum, penis, buccal mucosa, and in the umbilicus. They are individual, ectatic blood vessels covered with a few layers of skin. The lesions are without other symptoms, except that they have a tendency to bleed if traumatized. Corneal opacities are common but do not interfere with vision. Renal disease, coronary artery disease, and stroke occur in early adulthood. Autonomic nervous system dysfunction occurs and can present as chronic diarrhea, constipation, and the hypohidrosis described above. Cerebrovascular complications include hemiparesis, vertigo, diplopia, nystagmus, headache, ataxia, and memory loss.

Urine will show casts and Maltese crosses (birefringent lipid globules). Confirm diagnosis with finding deficiency of lysosomal α-galactosidase in plasma, leukocytes, or cultured skin fibroblasts.

Painful peripheral neuropathy may respond to carbamazepine or gabapentin. IV infusion of purified α-galactosidase may also relieve pain. Enzyme-replacement therapy is now clinically available and approved by the FDA. However, treatment of children and females remains controversial about when to start and why. Renal transplant is required for end-stage renal disease.

Sphingolipidoses: Important Things to Review

Let's review this difficult topic for things you really should know. All are AR, except for Fabry disease (X-linked). See Table 10-5 to help you remember which involve the CNS. Enzyme replacement is effective in preventing/reversing the hematologic and early skeletal complications of Gaucher (all types), but will not affect the neurologic problems of Types 2 and 3.

notes

PEROXISOMAL DISORDERS
OVERVIEW

First, what the heck are peroxisomes? These are organelles that have a single membrane and are found in just about all cells except RBCs. Peroxisomes contain > 50 different enzymes, including a group of important enzymes that catabolize β-oxidation of fatty acids. These are different from the enzymes in the mitochondria that do this. The peroxisomal enzymes oxidize very long- and long-chain fatty acids, while the mitochondrial enzymes oxidize the long-, medium-, and short-chain fatty acids. Another difference is that in peroxisomal oxidation, the first step is the production of hydrogen peroxide (H_2O_2), which is later eliminated by another enzyme in the peroxisomal cascade.

Generally, there are two classes of peroxisomal disorders:

1) Peroxisomal biogenesis disorders, which involve a deficiency of multiple peroxisome functions; and

2) Single-function disorders, in which only one peroxisomal function is missing

The peroxisomal biogenesis disorders are all AR, and their combined frequency for the 12+ disorders is about 1/50,000. Zellweger syndrome is the classic one usually described. The single-function peroxisome disorders are much less common and can be AR or X-linked in inheritance. The most commonly described is the X-linked adrenal leukodystrophy (X-ALD).

ZELLWEGER SYNDROME SPECTRUM

These are at the severe end of the spectrum for disorders of peroxisome function; this includes infantile Refsum disease and neonatal adrenoleukodystrophy. Onset of symptoms ranges from birth to 1–2 years of age with loss of skills and a progressive course. These infants have a characteristic facies with high forehead, epicanthal folds, broad-based nasal bridge, anteverted nares, and micrognathia. Other prominent findings include a large anterior fontanelle, cataracts, and pigmented retinopathy, hearing loss, and vision loss. Liver function is abnormal and jaundice occurs. Calcific stippling (discrete, precise calcifications) of the patella and epiphyses of the long bones is common. Most die before 1 year of age. Confirm diagnosis by looking for abnormalities of very long-chain fatty acids.

X-LINKED ADRENOLEUKODYSTROPHY (X-ALD)

There are multiple clinical presentations for boys with X-ALD. Most severe is the childhood cerebral form. It rapidly progresses with central demyelination and begins between 3 and 10 years of age. The childhood cerebral form occurs in > 33% of those affected and eventually progresses to death. Almost all of these boys have adrenal insufficiency. Another phenotype is adrenomyeloneuropathy (AMN). It doesn't show up until the 30s and 40s and presents with distal axonopathy of the spinal cord, causing gait disturbance and urinary sphincter dysfunction. ~ 66% have adrenal insufficiency, and nearly 40% will have cerebral effects.

Diagnosis is aided by looking for elevated plasma very long-chain fatty acid levels, particularly C26:0.

VARIOUS INHERITED DISORDERS WITH DYSMORPHIC FINDINGS
MENKES DISEASE (KINKY HAIR DISEASE)

This is a rare X-linked disease due to a mutation in the Menkes (*MNK*) gene, which causes impaired uptake of copper. It occurs in about 1/50,000–1/250,000 births. Boys will usually present in the neonatal period with premature delivery, temperature instability, hypothermia, hypotonia, and hypoglycemia. They have characteristic facies: pudgy cheeks and sagging jowls and lips. Hair and eyebrows are sparse with little pigment and are easily broken. We call it "kinky hair" disease because, under the microscope, the hair has "pili torti." By age 2–3 months, the child will have progressive neurologic deterioration, along with seizures and loss of milestones if he ever made any developmental gains. Collagen and bone formation are abnormal. This is one of the few genetic diseases that can have subdural hematomas and retinal hemorrhages not due to child abuse. It usually progresses, with death at ~ 2 years of age. Diagnosis is clinical and aided by finding low serum copper and ceruloplasmin levels after the first week of life. Copper measurements are high in intestinal biopsies but low in liver biopsies. When considering the diagnosis in an infant, you cannot rely on copper and ceruloplasmin levels since they are

Table 10-5: Sphingolipidoses—CNS or NOT?
CNS Diseases
CNS only without visceral involvement: Tay-Sachs disease
CNS with hepatosplenomegaly: Gaucher disease, Types 2 and 3 Niemann-Pick disease, Types A and C
CNS with cardiac, renal, vascular, or pulmonary: Niemann-Pick disease, Type A
Non-CNS Diseases
Predominantly hepatosplenomegaly: Gaucher disease, Type 1 Niemann-Pick disease, Type B
Peripheral nervous system with +/− skin lesions, cardiac, renal, vascular, or pulmonary: Fabry disease

notes

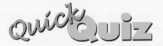

Quick Quiz

1) What metal has impaired utilization in Menkes disease?
2) What is Smith-Lemli-Opitz syndrome?
3) What is a common finding in most hepatic porphyrias?
4) Which drugs may "set off" acute intermittent porphyria?

normally low. You need to measure amounts of copper-containing compounds like dopamine.

SMITH-LEMLI-OPITZ SYNDROME

This is an AR disorder due to a defect in cholesterol biosynthesis. A deficient activity of 7-dehydrocholesterol reductase, it occurs in about 1/20,000–1/40,000 births. Remember: Cholesterol is very important in embryogenesis. Therefore, if abnormalities occur during this time, expect marked dysmorphology. The clinical range goes from an isolated 2/3-toe syndactyly with developmental delay to severely malformed fetuses that die *in utero*.

The characteristic facial features of the severe form include:

- Microcephaly
- Broad nasal tip
- Hypertelorism
- Cleft palate
- Micrognathia
- Anteverted nostrils
- Ptosis
- Low-set ears
- Narrow bifrontal diameter
- Abnormal thumbs

See Figure 10-4. You may also see postaxial polydactyly, overlapping fingers, and partial 2/3-toe syndactyly, as well as hypospadias and ambiguous genitalia. All organ systems may be affected, and mental retardation is standard. Congenital heart defects are common and should be investigated.

Serum levels of 7-dehydrocholesterol will be elevated, and cholesterol will be normal to low. (Remember: The enzyme is deficient, so you get a "backup" of 7-dehydrocholesterol, and the cholesterol level will inversely correlate with severity of disease.) Treatment with dietary cholesterol and bile-acid supplements to correct serum-cholesterol levels may be helpful.

PORPHYRIAS

OVERVIEW

These are a group of disorders caused by an enzyme defect in the heme synthesis pathway. Most base their classifications on whether the disorders are hepatic or erythropoietic in their overproduction and accumulation of the porphyrin precursor or the porphyrins. Generally, if it is hepatic in nature, you'll see neurologic abnormalities of neuropathy, mental disturbances, and abdominal pain, while the erythropoietic group will have cutaneous photosensitivity.

HEPATIC PORPHYRIAS

Acute Intermittent Porphyria

This is an AD disorder seen most commonly in Scandinavians and the British. It is due to a deficiency (usually about 1/2 normal) of HMB-synthetase (also known as PBG-deaminase or uroporphyrinogen I synthetase). Phenotypic expression is variable. Most heterozygotes are asymptomatic, unless some factor increases the production of pyrogens. The factors are varied and include endogenous and exogenous gonadal steroids, drugs, alcohol, and low-calorie diets.

The most common drugs on the Board exam to look for are:

- Barbiturates (phenobarbital)
- Sulfonamide antibiotics
- Anti-seizure medications, such as carbamazepine and valproic acid
- Griseofulvin
- Synthetic estrogens (birth control pills)

Note: Aspirin, phenothiazines, glucocorticoids, insulin, and acetaminophen are not likely to cause problems.

Abdominal pain is the most common symptom, along with ileus, abdominal distention, and decreased bowel sounds. Abdominal tenderness and fever are absent because this is a neurologic phenomenon, not inflammatory. Patients may also complain of nausea and vomiting with pain in the limbs, neck, or chest. Dysuria and urinary retention also occur.

Peripheral neuropathy is due to axonal degeneration and initially affects motor neurons of the proximal muscles of the shoulders and arms in particular. Sensory changes are less prominent than the motor dysfunction. Progressive weakness without effective treatment can lead to respiratory and bulbar paralysis. Mental symptoms are common, including anxiety, insomnia, depression, and paranoia during the acute attacks. Seizures may occur, which are complicated by the fact that anti-seizure medications will induce attacks. Bromides and

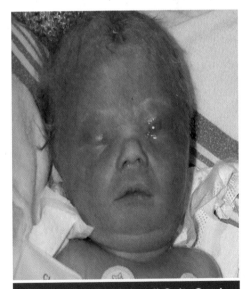

Figure 10-4: Smith-Lemli-Opitz Synd.

notes

clonazepam are probably the safest. Hyponatremia occurs because of hypothalamic involvement or SIADH.
After an attack, the abdominal pain will resolve in a few hours. The muscle weakness will improve over several days but may take years to return to normal.

You can best determine diagnosis by measuring hydroxymethyl biline (HMB) synthetase in RBCs; you also can screen asymptomatic family members. A normal PBG (porphobilinogen) level in the stool rules out acute intermittent porphyria.

You can treat acute attacks with narcotic analgesics for the abdominal pain, and phenothiazines may be helpful for nausea and vomiting. IV glucose (300 g/day) can be helpful in acute attacks, with continuous parenteral infusion if the patient cannot maintain oral intake. IV heme is probably the most effective therapy if given early. Infuse 4 grams of heme (usually as heme albumin or heme arginate) daily for 4 days, as soon as an attack begins. Some women have cyclical attacks, which can be prevented with a luteinizing hormone-releasing hormone analog.

Porphyria Cutanea Tarda (PCT)

Porphyria cutanea tarda (PCT) is the most common of the porphyrias. There are 4 types: Type I—sporadic; Types II and III—familial; and Type IV—occurs after exposure to halogenated, aromatic hydrocarbons. The defect in all types is a deficiency of hepatic URO-decarboxylase. Type I has normal levels in RBCs. Type II is deficient in RBCs and other tissues. Type III is deficient only in the liver. The hydrocarbon-induced form occurs in normal individuals and results from a decrease in enzymes in the liver on exposure to the hydrocarbon.

Patients present with cutaneous photosensitivity and develop fluid-filled vesicles and bullae on the sun-exposed areas of the face, the dorsa of the hands and feet, the forearms, and the legs. Milia may precede or follow the vesicles. Hypertrichosis and hyperpigmentation are also common.
Excess alcohol, iron, and estrogen can contribute to the development of hepatic URO-decarboxylase deficiency. Drugs also have been implicated, including accidental exposure to the fungicide hexachlorobenzene, dioxin, and chlorophenols.

Patients usually have liver damage and are predisposed to develop hepatocellular carcinoma.
Finding increased porphyrin levels in liver, plasma, urine, and stool helps with diagnosis. Types II and III can be diagnosed by finding decreased URO-decarboxylase activity in RBCs.
Aim treatment at preventing exposure to the offending agent. Usually, you can obtain complete response by phlebotomy to reduce hepatic iron. A unit of blood (450 mL) can be removed every 1–2 weeks. Usually, remission will occur after 5 or 6 phlebotomies. After remission, some will stay well while others will require repeated phlebotomies. You can also treat PCT with chloroquine or hydroxychloroquine.

These complex with excess porphyrins, and enhance excretion. Give only small doses (125 mg), because larger doses may precipitate an acute attack.

ERYTHROPOIETIC PORPHYRIAS

X-linked Sideroblastic Anemia

This is due to deficient activity of the erythroid form of aminolevulinate (ALA) synthase and is associated with ineffective erythropoiesis and weakness. Infant boys will develop refractory hemolytic anemia, pallor, and weakness. Secondary hypersplenism is common. Blood smears show hypochromic, microcytic anemia with anisocytosis (cells of many different sizes), poikilocytosis (irregular shapes), and polychromasia (different colors). WBCs and platelets are normal. Hemoglobin is reduced, and MCV and MCHC are both decreased.
Bone marrow studies will show a hypercellular marrow with megaloblastic erythropoieses. Sideroblasts are commonly seen. Urinary porphyrin and its precursors are normal. Definitive diagnosis is finding the mutations in the erythroid ALA synthase gene.
Anemia may respond to pyridoxine (B_6). Those who don't respond require transfusions and long-term chelation therapy.

Erythropoietic Protoporphyria (EPP)

EPP is an AD disease that is due to a partial deficiency of ferrochelatase. Protoporphyrin accumulates abnormally in erythroid cells and plasma and is excreted in bile and feces. This is the most common erythropoietic porphyria and is second behind porphyria cutanea tarda for all porphyrias.

Skin photosensitivity is the major clinical feature and begins in childhood. It is different from the other porphyrias in that vesicles are not common—and pigment changes, severe scarring, and hirsutism are unusual. It looks more like angioedema, and, within minutes of sun exposure, patients will have redness, burning, itching, and swelling.
The source of the excess protoporphyrin is the bone marrow reticulocyte. Liver function is usually normal; but occasionally, chronic liver disease will develop. Gallstones can also occur and will contain protoporphyrin.

Finding elevated levels of protoporphyrin in bone marrow, RBCs, plasma, bile, and feces is diagnostic. Urinary levels of porphyrin and its precursors are normal. Ferrochelatase activity is decreased in fibroblasts.

Oral beta-carotene improves tolerance to sunlight. Hepatic complications are more difficult to treat. Cholestyramine and activated charcoal may cause the interruption of protoporphyrin circulation and lead to its excretion in the feces. Splenectomy can be helpful for those with significant splenomegaly. Transfusions and IV heme may be helpful in suppressing protoporphyrin production. A few patients with severe liver dysfunction have received liver transplants.

notes

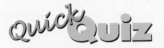

Quick Quiz

1) How do children with porphyria cutanea tarda present?

2) What therapy will result in remission of porphyria cutanea tarda?

3) How does an individual with X-linked sideroblastic anemia present?

4) How does a child with EPP present?

5) How may a child with adenylate deaminase deficiency present?

6) Describe Lesch-Nyhan disease.

7) What do you look for in homozygotes with familial hypercholesterolemia?

8) What disease should you suspect in a child whose 3 uncles and his father all have tendon xanthomas?

9) What complaints would you expect from a child with excessive chylomicronemia? If you draw blood from an affected child, spin it down, and leave the plasma in a test tube unaffected overnight, what will you see in the morning?

PURINE DISORDERS

PHOSPHORIBOSYL PYROPHOSPHATE SYNTHETASE SUPERACTIVITY

This is a rare X-linked disorder and causes gout. A severe phenotype with gout, neurodevelopmental delay, and sensorineural deafness occurs in young children. Allopurinol is effective.

ADENYLATE DEAMINASE DEFICIENCY

This is an AR trait that occurs in 1–2% of the population. It presents as muscle weakness and cramping following vigorous exercise. Serum CK may be increased, but myoglobinuria is not associated with this deficiency. Muscle biopsy is normal. A specific histochemical stain is necessary for diagnosis, and many with the deficiency are asymptomatic.

LESCH-NYHAN DISEASE
(Hypoxanthine Guanine Phosphoribosyltransferase [HGPRT] Deficiency)

Lesch-Nyhan disease is an X-linked disorder due to deficiency of HGPRT. This enzyme preserves hypoxanthine and guanine, then converts them to nucleotides. Males are normal at birth but by age 3–6 months have FTT, emesis, and irritability. By age 2–3 years, self-mutilation, the most disturbing

manifestation, develops. The children bite their lips and fingers. Renal stones and gout occur because of the huge increase in uric acid production.

You can diagnose HGPRT deficiency in red blood cells and cultured skin fibroblasts.

DISORDERS OF LIPIDS AND LIPOPROTEINS

NOTE

Screening guidelines are discussed in Growth and Development /Preventive Pediatrics section.

HYPERLIPOPROTEINEMIA DISORDERS

Familial Hypercholesterolemia (FH)

Familial hypercholesterolemia (FH) occurs in 1/200–1/500. The disorder is due to > 150 different mutations at the gene locus for LDL receptor protein. Familial hypercholesterolemia is AD in its transmission. Heterozygous children are usually asymptomatic in the first decade but, by the second decade, nearly 10–15% develop xanthomas of the Achilles or extensor hand tendons.

Achillis tendinitis or tenosynovitis may be the first clue in a teenage patient. Homozygous children develop planar xanthomas (flat, orange-colored skin lesions) from birth to age 5 years.

Serum cholesterol is usually 600–1,000 mg/dL. Tendon and tuberous xanthomas occur in ages 5–15 years. Angina and symptomatic coronary disease occur in the second decade and have been documented in those < 10 years of age.

Untreated FH male heterozygotes have a 100% risk of developing coronary heart disease by age 70, while untreated females have a 75% risk. Treatment reduces this risk by normalizing cholesterol.

Look for a child with parents who have tendon xanthomas or a large number of 1st degree relatives with highly elevated LDL cholesterol levels. Be aware that other conditions can cause lipid deposition, such as biliary cirrhosis, congenital biliary atresia, myelomas, and Wolman disease; but other findings also will be apparent to help you differentiate between them.

Be on the lookout for sitosterolemia, a rare inherited plant sterol storage disease. This disorder has tendon xanthomas in the first decade but only moderate hypercholesterolemia.

notes

Familial Combined Hyperlipidemia

Familial combined hyperlipidemia is a syndrome where LDL is usually elevated, but the LDL receptor activity is normal. The increased LDL is due to overproduction of VLDL and apoB in the liver. It occurs in ~ 1/100. These children can have elevated LDL alone (Type IIa), elevated LDL and triglyceride (Type IIb), or normal LDL and elevated triglyceride (Type IV). This presents in adults with early coronary artery disease. Corneal arcus may occur, but xanthomas do not.

Hyperapobetalipoproteinemia

Hyperapobetalipoproteinemia has a characteristic elevated LDL apoB level with a normal LDL level, while triglycerides can be normal or elevated. It is due to overproduction of VLDL.

Familial Hypertriglyceridemia

These children will have normal total cholesterol and LDL levels, but will have elevated VLDL and triglyceride levels (Type IV pattern).

Lipoprotein-lipase Deficiency

Lipoprotein-lipase enzyme deficiency/defectiveness results in huge increases of chylomicrons with marked hypertriglyceridemia (up to 10,000 mg/dL). Marked chylomicronemia usually indicates that the body cannot clear dietary fat. You can demonstrate this by leaving an affected individual's plasma in a test tube overnight. In the morning, you will see a thick, creamy layer. VLDL is normal, and LDL and HDL are low. It will usually occur/present before 10 years of age with abdominal pain as the initial complaint; colic, in particular, will occur in infants < 1 year. Eruptive xanthomas, hepatosplenomegaly, and retinal deposits may occur; atherosclerosis usually does not.

Type V Hyperlipoproteinemia

These patients have a marked triglyceride level due to increased chylomicrons and VLDL. Pancreatitis, eruptive xanthomas, and hyperinsulinemia are common. AD inheritance has been shown in a large number of these cases.

Dysbetalipoproteinemia (Type III)

These patients have elevated cholesterol and triglyceride levels. Characteristic for this syndrome is plasma VLDL that is cholesterol-enriched and has β, rather than pre-β, electrophoresis. This disease usually doesn't manifest until adulthood, with xanthomas in the creases of the palms and tuberous xanthomas of the elbows, knees, and buttocks. Premature atherosclerosis is common, although tendon xanthomas are not.

HYPOLIPOPROTEINEMIA DISORDERS

Abetalipoproteinemia (Bassen-Kornzweig Syndrome)

This is a rare AR disorder, which presents in children with fat malabsorption, hypolipidemia, retinitis pigmentosa, cerebellar ataxia, and acanthocytosis. Chylomicrons, VLDL, and LDL are absent from plasma. Cholesterol and triglycerides are low. Diagnosis: jejunal biopsy, failure to form chylomicrons after a fatty meal, or demonstrating the absence of apoprotein B in plasma. Clinically, this is important because the fat-soluble vitamins (A, D, E, and K) are dependent and cannot be absorbed or transported properly. However, only vitamin E deficiency is clinically apparent because of other transport mechanisms available. The retinal and nervous system effects are due to vitamin E deficiency.

Tangier Disease

This is a rare disorder in which plasma HDL is abnormal and deficient. Cholesterol ester is deposited in tissues, resulting in enlarged, orange-yellow tonsils, splenomegaly, and peripheral neuropathy.

NEWBORN SCREENING (NBS)

More and more inborn errors of metabolism are detected by the newborn heel stick. What was once known as the "PKU" test now covers about 36 disorders in the majority of states. It is important you know which disorders discussed above could be detected on newborn screening (NBS).

You don't need an overview of NBS philosophy, but you should have an idea of why some disorders (as opposed to others) are part of the screen. The idea of NBS is to detect life-threatening and/or potentially serious disorders that can be treated effectively.

At this time, the disorders we screen for are limited to defects causing intoxications and/or energy metabolism defects. So what is covered?
- Amino acid defects
- Fatty acid oxidation defects
- Galactosemia
- Biotinidase deficiency

Non-metabolic disorders on NBS are:
- Hemoglobinopathies
- Endocrine disorders, such as congenital adrenal hyperplasia and congenital hypothyroidism
- Cystic fibrosis

Not covered are storage disorders, complex molecule defects, or mitochondrial defects.

MedStudy®

4th Edition

Pediatrics Board Review Core Curriculum

Neurology

Authored by J. Thomas Cross, Jr., MD, MPH, FAAP, and Robert A. Hannaman, MD

Many thanks to

Patricia K. Duffner, MD
Professor of Neurology and Pediatrics
Department of Neurology
SUNY at Buffalo School of Medicine
Children's Hospital
Buffalo, NY

Neurology Advisor

Table of Contents

Neurology

CONGENITAL ANOMALIES OF THE CENTRAL
NERVOUS SYSTEM 11-1
  PREVENTION OF NEURAL TUBE DEFECTS 11-1
  ANENCEPHALY... 11-1
  ENCEPHALOCELE 11-1
  HYDROCEPHALUS 11-1
    What Is Hydrocephalus? 11-1
    Noncommunicating vs. Communicating....................... 11-1
    Anatomy Review 11-1
    Basic Plumbing 11-2
    Causes of Hydrocephalus 11-2
    Symptoms and Signs of Hydrocephalus 11-2
    Treatment of Hydrocephalus 11-2
  HYDROMELIA 11-3
  SYRINGOMYELIA.. 11-3
  SPINA BIFIDA OCCULTA 11-3
  MENINGOCELE 11-4
  MYELOMENINGOCELE 11-4
    Overview 11-4
    Clinical Findings 11-4
    Treatment of Myelomeningocele 11-4
  CHIARI (ARNOLD-CHIARI) MALFORMATION.................. 11-5
  KLIPPEL-FEIL SYNDROME 11-5
  LISSENCEPHALY (AGYRIA) 11-6
  SCHIZENCEPHALY 11-6
  PORENCEPHALY 11-6
  HOLOPROSENCEPHALY 11-6
  AGENESIS OF THE CORPUS CALLOSUM 11-6
CEREBRAL PALSY 11-7
  DEFINITIONS 11-7
  ETIOLOGY 11-7
    The Bottom Line.. 11-7
    Asphyxia 11-7
    Low Birth Weight 11-7
    Congenital Malformations.. 11-7
    Infection 11-7
    Inflammatory Mediators 11-7
  SPASTIC CP 11-8
  DYSKINETIC CP 11-8
  ATAXIC CP 11-8
  MIXED FORMS 11-8
  SEIZURES AND MENTAL RETARDATION 11-8
  DIAGNOSIS OF CP... 11-8
  TREATMENT OF CP 11-8
CEREBROVASCULAR DISEASES 11-8
  OVERVIEW 11-8
  MAJOR CAUSES OF ISCHEMIC STROKES IN
    CHILDREN 11-9
    Cardiac Disorders 11-9
    Prothrombotic Disorders 11-9
    Sickle-cell Disease 11-9
    Cervicocephalic Arterial Dissection 11-9
    CNS Vasculitis 11-10
    Metabolic Etiologies... 11-10
  NEONATAL CEREBRAL INFARCTION 11-10
  HEMORRHAGIC STROKE... 11-10
  CEREBRAL VEIN THROMBOSIS 11-11
INJURY / TRAUMA TO THE CENTRAL AND
PERIPHERAL NERVOUS SYSTEMS 11-11
  OCCURRENCE 11-11
  SCALP INJURIES 11-11
    Lacerations... 11-11
    Hematomas 11-11

    Skull Fractures 11-12
  PARENCHYMAL INJURIES 11-12
    Cerebral Contusion 11-12
    Diffuse Axonal Injury... 11-12
    Epidural Hematoma.. 11-12
    Subdural Hematoma 11-13
  SPINAL CORD INJURY 11-13
  COMMON PERIPHERAL NERVE INJURIES...................... 11-14
    Birth Trauma 11-14
    Erb-Duchenne Type Injuries (Upper Plexus Root)............ 11-14
    Klumpke-Dejerine Type Injuries (Lower Plexus Root)...... 11-14
    Serratus Anterior Palsy 11-14
    Sciatic Nerve Injury 11-14
SEIZURE DISORDERS.. 11-14
  OCCURRENCE 11-14
  PRIMARY GENERALIZED SEIZURES 11-14
    Mechanism / Characteristics 11-14
    Tonic-Clonic Seizures (Grand Mal Seizure) 11-15
    Myoclonic Seizures 11-15
    Juvenile Myoclonic Epilepsy (Janz Syndrome) 11-15
    Absence Seizures (Petit Mal Seizures)........................... 11-15
    Atonic or Akinetic Seizures (Epileptic Drop Attacks)........ 11-16
  PARTIAL (FOCAL) SEIZURES 11-16
    Occurrence 11-16
    Simple Partial Seizures 11-16
    Complex Partial Seizures 11-16
  INFANTILE SPASMS (WEST SYNDROME)....................... 11-16
  LENNOX-GASTAUT SYNDROME 11-17
  POST-TRAUMATIC SEIZURES....................................... 11-17
  OTHER SEIZURE TYPES 11-17
    Flickering-Light or Video Game-Induced Seizures 11-17
    Acquired Epileptic Aphasia (Landau-Kleffner Syndrome) 11-17
    Epilepsia Partialis Continua..................................... 11-17
    Rasmussen Syndrome 11-17
    Other Seizures 11-18
  DRUG THERAPY AND SIDE EFFECTS 11-18
    Valproate (Valproic Acid) 11-18
    Carbamazepine 11-18
    Phenytoin 11-18
    Ethosuximide 11-18
    Phenobarbital 11-18
    Oxcarbazepine 11-18
    Lamotrigine 11-18
  STATUS EPILEPTICUS... 11-18
  COMMON EPILEPSY QUESTIONS 11-19
    When to Stop Therapy? 11-19
    What Are the Teratogenic Effects of These Drugs? 11-19
    What about Breastfeeding?.. 11-19
  NEONATAL SEIZURES 11-19
  FEBRILE SEIZURES 11-20
MIGRAINE HEADACHES 11-21
NEUROMUSCULAR DISEASES 11-22
  SPINAL MUSCULAR ATROPHY 11-22
  DUCHENNE MUSCULAR DYSTROPHY 11-22
  MYASTHENIA GRAVIS 11-22
  GUILLAIN-BARRÉ SYNDROME 11-23
  BOTULISM 11-23
MISCELLANEOUS DISORDERS.. 11-24
  NOTE 11-24
  ACUTE CEREBELLAR ATAXIA OF CHILDHOOD............ 11-24
  TRANSVERSE MYELITIS 11-24
  MULTIPLE SCLEROSIS 11-24

CONGENITAL ANOMALIES OF THE CENTRAL NERVOUS SYSTEM

PREVENTION OF NEURAL TUBE DEFECTS

Folic acid supplements reduce the risk of neural tube defects. In 2009, the U.S. Preventive Services Task Force (USPSTF) recommended that all women of reproductive age consume 0.4 to 0.8 mg of folic acid daily (0.4 mg is the usual dose in over-the-counter multivitamins). The AAP recommends that women with a previously affected child and those on anticonvulsant drugs take 4.0 mg of folic acid daily beginning 1 month before conception and continuing through the 1st trimester.

ANENCEPHALY

Anencephaly occurs with an incidence of ~ 1/10,000 live births (a rate that underestimates the actual rate due to spontaneous abortion and pregnancy termination) and is incompatible with survival. Girls are more commonly affected than boys and Caucasians more commonly than African-Americans. It occurs due to failure of closure of the anterior neural tube (neuropore). (Failure of closure of the posterior neuropore results in myelomeningocele.) Those affected have large parts of the cranium missing, especially the frontal, parietal, and occipital bones. It always involves the forebrain and can also extend to the base. Usually, there is no hypothalamus. Associated malformations of the face and eyes are common. The hypoplastic pituitary gland causes failure of end-organ development, leading, for example, to adrenal insufficiency.

Suspect anencephaly prenatally if you find elevated maternal serum levels of α-fetoprotein. Fetal ultrasound will confirm the diagnosis.

ENCEPHALOCELE

An encephalocele is a herniation of the brain, its coverings, or both, through a skull defect; 75% of the time, it is in the occipital region. It occurs in ~ 1–2/10,000 live births but is less common than anencephaly in its total incidence due to the high number of spontaneous abortions/terminations in anencephaly. Males and females are equally affected. The herniated materials can contain meninges, cerebrospinal fluid (CSF), or dysplastic neural tissue. The size of the sac does not correlate with the amount of brain tissue present; transillumination will give a better idea. If just meninges are in the sac, many do well with normal development, without central nervous system (CNS) defects. Obviously, significant brain tissue involvement will affect the severity of the lesion. Use CT/MRI to determine the extent of brain tissue in the encephalocele. Prenatal diagnosis may be confirmed by ultrasound, and also you can see an elevated α-fetoprotein (but if the defect is covered by skin/scalp the level can be normal). Treatment: Remove the sac and close the defect as early as possible.

HYDROCEPHALUS

What Is Hydrocephalus?

Hydrocephalus is not a specific disease, but rather describes a diverse group of disorders that result from impaired circulation and CSF absorption or, rarely, from increased CSF production, usually by a choroid plexus papilloma. The absorption of CSF is inhibited by either mechanical or functional blockage of the flow of fluid along its usual path. With this blockage, there is increased pressure in the ventricular system.

Noncommunicating vs. Communicating

Hydrocephalus can be either noncommunicating or communicating. Noncommunicating refers to the accumulation of ventricular fluid, wherein the fluid does not communicate with CSF in the spinal subarachnoid spaces or in the basal cisterns. A noncommunicating hydrocephalus is due to a block of CSF flow somewhere in the ventricular system, most commonly in the foramen of Monro, the aqueduct of Sylvius, or the 4th ventricle and its outlets. A communicating hydrocephalus is due to blockage of CSF flow outside of the ventricular system, wherein the ventricular fluid communicates with the spinal subarachnoid space and basal cisterns. Complete blockage of, or complete inability to absorb, CSF is incompatible with life in the absence of shunting procedures.

Anatomy Review

The choroid plexus produces CSF. Each of the 4 ventricles contains choroid plexus tissue.

Let's review the normal anatomy of how the ventricular system connects:
Paired lateral ventricles → paired foramen of Monro → single midline 3rd ventricle → aqueduct of Sylvius → midline 4th ventricle → 3 exit openings: paired lateral foramina of Luschka and a midline foramen of Magendie → spinal subarachnoid space → intracranial subarachnoid space over the cerebral convexities → absorbed into the venous sinuses via the arachnoid granulations.
In the ventricular system, CSF flows as follows:
Lateral ventricles → 3rd ventricle → 4th ventricle → basal cisterns → tentorium → subarachnoid space → arachnoid granulations → venous sinuses.
In the spinal subarachnoid space, the fluid flows toward the head.

Most of the CSF is absorbed by the arachnoid granulations (over the convexities) and in the spinal subarachnoid space. Less fluid is absorbed by the ependyma of the ventricular system. In an adult, the normal CSF volume is 150 mL with 25% within the ventricular system. CSF can be formed at a rate of 20 mL/hour. Thus, we know that CSF is "turned over" 3–4 times a day.

notes

Basic Plumbing

Obstruction of CSF flow is the most common cause of hydrocephalus. Hydrocephalus is defined as an excessive volume of intracranial cerebrospinal fluid. Think of hydrocephalus as a plumbing problem, and review the "plumbing" noted above—because proximal to the blockage, the ventricular system will dilate and expand. For example: If one foramen of Monro is obstructed, the lateral ventricle on that side will dilate. If the aqueduct of Sylvius is obstructed, will the 4th ventricle be enlarged? No, because that ventricle is after the obstruction. In communicating hydrocephalus (remember this is outside the ventricular system), the whole ventricular system is dilated!

Excessive CSF production is rare and may be associated with functional choroid plexus papillomas and carcinomas. Surgical removal may cure the hydrocephalus; but because of the highly vascular nature of the tumor, the associated bleeding may cause communicating hydrocephalus due to poor absorption of the CSF into the venous system. Sometimes, the tumor will also cause a noncommunicating hydrocephalus if it obstructs the foramen of Monro or the 4th ventricle.

Causes of Hydrocephalus

There are many causes for hydrocephalus. Most texts separate causes of hydrocephalus based on the terms "communicating" and "noncommunicating."

The most common causes of communicating hydrocephalus are meningitis and subarachnoid hemorrhage. Meningeal leukemia may also reduce resorption of CSF. Communicating hydrocephalus can develop from an infection of the CNS—especially bacterial meningitis and mumps. Hydrocephalus can be due to intrauterine infection, such as CMV, rubella, toxoplasmosis, and syphilis. These infections cause an inflammatory reaction of the ependymal linings of the ventricular system and the meninges of the subarachnoid space, resulting in decreased ability to absorb CSF.

Noncommunicating hydrocephalus results in the occlusion of the CSF pathway and can be either acquired (posterior fossa tumors) or congenital. An example is obstruction in the aqueduct of Sylvius or basal cisterns, which can occur with congenital aqueductal stenosis. The Dandy-Walker malformation consists of a posterior fossa cyst that is continuous with the 4th ventricle, partial or complete absence of the cerebellar vermis, and hydrocephalus. The Chiari malformation occurs when parts of the brainstem and cerebellum are displaced down into the cervical spinal canal, and the flow of spinal fluid is impaired in the posterior fossa. This malformation is associated with hydrocephalus, spina bifida, and meningomyelocele. There is also a sex-linked, genetic form of congenital hydrocephalus due to aqueductal stenosis.

Acquired causes that obstruct the intraventricular pathway include brain tumors, intraventricular clots, abscess, and vein of Galen malformation.

Symptoms and Signs of Hydrocephalus

Many of the symptoms and signs are due to the underlying cause of the hydrocephalus. Much depends on the rate of CSF accumulation and the pace of the hydrocephalus. If accumulation is slow, you may note few symptoms, while rapidly progressive ventricular dilatation produces symptoms quickly. Headaches are the most common, nonspecific symptom in older children. Early-morning headaches, along with nausea and vomiting, are often associated with hydrocephalus. Personality and behavior changes are common. If the midbrain or brain stem is involved, lethargy and drowsiness may occur. Increased intracranial pressure can result in papilledema and extraocular muscle palsies, especially involving the 3rd and 6th cranial nerves.

In time, bradycardia, systemic hypertension, and altered respiratory rates may occur if brainstem function is affected. In infants and young children, you may notice excessive head growth on serial examinations. "Frontal bossing" may occur in the infant, and scalp veins may dilate. "Setting sun sign" occurs when upward gaze is impaired because of pressure on the midbrain, and the sclera above the iris will become visible. Lower extremity spasticity, growth disturbances, early pubertal development, or fluid/electrolyte disorders also may occur.

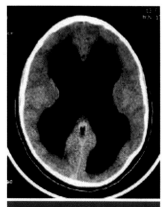

Figure 11-1: Hydrocephalus

You must conduct routine and serial head circumference measurements for diagnosis.

CT or MRI is diagnostic. (See Figure 11-1.)

Treatment of Hydrocephalus

Treat the underlying condition if possible. Surgical therapy is the most effective treatment for hydrocephalus. Usually, you would use a mechanical shunt system to circumvent the obstruction (See? It's back to plumbing). Place a catheter in the right lateral ventricle, and connect by a one-way valve system that opens when the pressure in the ventricle exceeds a predetermined baseline level. The valve is usually placed under the scalp, in the postauricular area. Then place the distal end in the right atrium (a ventriculoatrial shunt, less commonly used today) or into the peritoneal cavity (ventriculoperitoneal shunt, the majority today). If the shunt becomes obstructed or nonfunctioning, hydrocephalus can recur and symptoms will reappear. Shunt revision then likely will be necessary.

Diagnose intrauterine hydrocephalus with fetal ultrasound.

Besides the mechanical problems, shunts can become infected and result in ventriculitis. Shunt infection can be benign or severe. Many children will have fever and may have hydrocephalus symptoms if the shunt malfunctions. The most

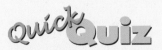
common organism responsible is *Staphylococcus epidermidis*, which usually responds only to vancomycin. Other less common organisms include *S. aureus*, *E. coli* and other Gram negatives, diphtheroids, and *Streptococcus* species. Some neurosurgeons will try to treat an infected shunt with antibiotics in an attempt to "clear it." This is rarely successful.

Another problem with ventriculoatrial shunts: They can lead to pulmonary hypertension if chronic microemboli occur from the atrial catheter.

You may attempt medical therapy if the hydrocephalus is slowly progressive and no signs/symptoms appear. Commonly used agents include acetazolamide and furosemide. But note: Medical therapy is not as good as surgical intervention.

HYDROMELIA

Hydromelia is a symmetric dilation of the central canal of the spinal cord by CSF and usually communicates with the 4th ventricle. It is lined with ependyma. Hydromelia is associated with communicating hydrocephalus, Chiari malformation, and aqueductal stenosis. Symptoms, when present, are usually related to the associated malformations. The hydromelia itself frequently does not cause any problems.

MRI makes the diagnosis. Treatment is rarely necessary for the dilation itself.

SYRINGOMYELIA

Syringomyelia is relatively rare and presents as a paracentral cavity, known as a syrinx, in the spinal cord. The cavity is lined with abnormal glial elements. The syrinx can be localized or involve multiple segments, especially in the cervical spine. If the lesion extends up to the brainstem, it is known as syringobulbia. The fluid in the cyst is yellowish. There is a strong association with Chiari I.

Symptoms depend on where the syrinx is located. Wasting of the small muscles of the hand, sensory deficits of the arms, or absence of deep tendon reflexes are common. Damage to crossing sensory fibers (lateral spinothalamic tracts) results in bilateral loss of pain and temperature sensation, leading to trophic ulcers of the finger tips. Respiratory problems in sleep are also common in those with syringobulbia.

MRI makes the diagnosis. (See Figure 11-2.) Treat by correcting malformations and/or performing myelotomy. Posterior fossa decompression is helpful in those patients who also have Chiari I malformation.

SPINA BIFIDA OCCULTA

Spina bifida occulta is a midline defect of the vertebral bodies without protrusion of the spinal cord or meninges. Most are asymptomatic and have no neurologic signs. Some cases present with patches of hair, a lipoma, skin-color changes, or a dermal sinus in the midline of the lower back, indicating the underlying spina bifida occulta. (See Figure 11-3.) Typically involved are L5 and S1, and plain x-rays of the spine show the defect. No treatment is necessary for most cases.

Occasionally, spina bifida occulta is associated with other spinal cord problems, including syringomyelia, diastematomyelia, or a tethered cord (abnormally low position of the spinal cord due to aberrant nerve roots or fibrous bands adhering to nervous tissue from the bony canal).

A dermoid sinus may occur and presents as a small skin opening leading into a narrow duct below the skin. It sometimes has protruding hairs, a hairy patch, or a vascular nevus on the surface. Dermoid sinuses can occur in the lumbar region, indicating meningoceles (described below) or in the occipital region, indicating encephaloceles (described above). Sometimes, the sinuses pass through the dura and result in recurrent infections, such as meningitis.

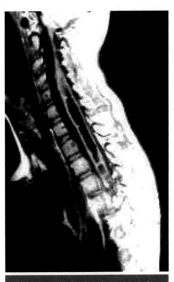

Figure 11-2: Syringomyelia

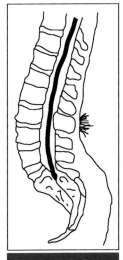

Figure 11-3: Spina Bifida Occulta

notes

MENINGOCELE

A meningocele refers to a herniation of the meninges through a defect in the posterior vertebral arches. (See Figure 11-4.) The spinal cord itself is usually normal. On transillumination along the vertebral column, you may see a fluctuant midline mass, usually in the low back. Most meningoceles are well covered with skin and pose no specific problem.

You can delay surgery in children with completely normal neurologic examinations and complete full-thickness skin covering of the meningocele. This scenario allows for full radiologic review to determine the extent of neurologic involvement for possible diastematomyelia (complete or incomplete sagittal division of the spinal cord by an osseous or fibrocartilaginous septum), tethered spinal cord, or lipomas.

Children with leaking CSF from the meningocele, or incomplete skin covering, need immediate surgical repair to prevent meningitis.

Sometimes, the meningocele can occur anteriorly and project into the pelvis through a defect in the sacrum. This protrusion may cause constipation and bladder dysfunction if it increases in size.

MYELOMENINGOCELE

Overview

Myelomeningocele (meningomyelocele, spina bifida) occurs in ~ 1–2/1,000 births and is the most severe form of neural tube defect involving the vertebral column. With one previously affected child, the risk in subsequent siblings increases to 3–4%; with 2 previously affected children, the subsequent sibling risk increases to 10%. There is very strong evidence that administration of folic acid before conception reduces the risk of spina bifida by > 50–60%. Give the folic acid before conception and during the first 12 weeks of gestation.

Today, most recommend that all women of childbearing potential take 0.4–0.8 mg of folic acid daily. A woman with a previously affected child with spina bifida should take 4.0 mg of folic acid, starting 1 month before attempting conception. Certain drugs increase the risk, especially valproic acid, which has a 1–2% risk of a neural tube defect.

Clinical Findings

A myelomeningocele involves the nerve roots, spinal cord meninges, vertebral bodies, and skin. (See Figure 11-5 and Figure 11-6.) It may be located anywhere along the neuro axis, but most commonly affects the lumbosacral region. The extent and degree of neurologic deficit depends on the location. For example: A low, sacral-region myelomeningocele will result in bowel and bladder incontinence and numbness of the perineal area but no motor dysfunction. Another example: Lower, lumbar myelomeningoceles present as sac-like cysts that are covered by a thin layer of partially epithelized tissue. In this location, the infant will have flaccid paralysis of the lower extremities, no deep tendon reflexes of the lower extremities, lack of response to touch or pain in the lower extremities, and postural abnormalities, such as clubfeet or hip subluxation. The child will have continuous, slow urine production, and the anal sphincter tone will be relaxed. Generally, as the lesion advances up the spine into the thoracic region, the more severe and extensive the neurologic manifestations will be. However, as the lesion continues into the upper thoracic or cervical areas, the neurologic manifestations are minimal and do not cause hydrocephalus!

Around 80–85% of children with myelomeningocele will develop hydrocephalus in addition to a Type II Chiari defect (see below). Again, as a general rule (except for thoracic/cervical areas), the lower down the spine the lesion is (e.g., sacrum), the less likely hydrocephalus will occur.

Treatment of Myelomeningocele

Treatment involves a multidisciplinary team with the pediatrician frequently acting as coordinator. You can delay repair of the myelomeningocele a few days if there is no CSF leak. After repair, most infants require a shunt for hydrocephalus. You must pay special attention to the GU system and bladder

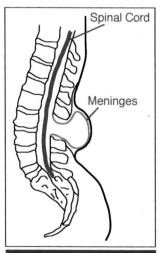

Figure 11-4: Meningocele

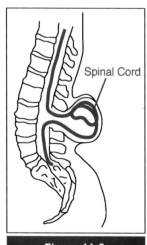

Figure 11-5: Myelomeningocele

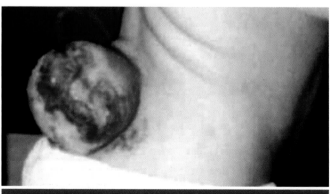

Figure 11-6: Myelomeningocele

notes

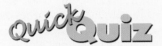

catheterization, because neurogenic bladder is common. Walking is possible for most children with sacral or lumbosacral lesions. For ~ 50% with higher lesions, use of a cane and brace will allow some ambulation. Prognosis for survival is generally good, with mortality rates ~ 15%; most deaths occur before age 4 years. ~ 75% of survivors have normal intelligence.

CHIARI (ARNOLD-CHIARI) MALFORMATION

Chiari (or Arnold-Chiari) malformation—not to be confused with Budd-Chiari syndrome, which is a hepatic blood flow obstruction—is a hindbrain abnormality, in which there is downward (caudal) displacement of the brainstem and cerebellum.

There are 3 types classified, based on the degree of displacement:

1) Type I: The cerebellar tonsils or vermis are pushed down below the level of the foramen magnum. (See Figure 11-7.) Generally, > 0.5 cm displacement is considered significant. Type I lesions can become symptomatic at any time between infancy and adulthood. Symptoms occur due to dysfunction of lower cranial nerves, the brainstem, and/or the spinal cord. These symptoms can include dysphagia, vertigo, sleep apnea, ataxia, headache, and neck pain. Spinal cord dysfunction may present as weakness, spasticity of the extremities, sensory loss, and occasionally, bowel and bladder dysfunction.

2) Type II: The most common form, which occurs when the 4th ventricle and lower medulla are pushed down below the level of the foramen magnum. Type II is almost always associated with myelomeningocele and hydrocephalus. Children with Type II are usually diagnosed at birth, and the symptoms relate to lower cranial nerve dysfunction. Patients with Type II have symptoms similar to those in Type I, but they have the added burden/symptoms of the accompanying hydrocephalus and myelomeningocele.

3) Type III: Herniation of the cerebellum occurs through a cervical spina bifida defect.

For asymptomatic Chiari I malformation, no treatment is necessary. Symptomatic children may benefit from surgery, including suboccipital decompressions with or without cervical laminectomies. Carefully discern if referred symptoms are indeed related to the malformation.

KLIPPEL-FEIL SYNDROME

Klippel-Feil syndrome has a classic triad of symptoms:
- short neck,
- limited neck motion, and
- low occipital hairline.

There are 3 types of Klippel-Feil syndrome, based on the extent of vertebral column malformation:

1) Type I—A majority of the cervical and upper thoracic vertebrae are fused into a "bony block."
2) Type II—"Complete" segmentation fails to occur at 1–2 cervical interspaces; this results in only a couple or several fused cervical vertebrae.
3) Type III—Similar lesions occur as above, but there are also segmentation errors in the lower thoracic and lumbar vertebrae.

Frequently, fusion of C2–3 is autosomal dominant (AD) in inheritance, while C5–6 is autosomal recessive (AR). Many other congenital anomalies are likely—including deafness, macrocephaly, hydrocephalus, meningocele, and mental

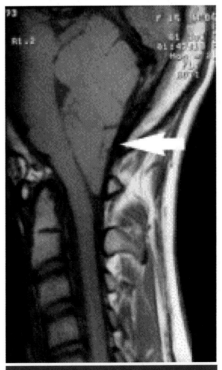

Figure 11-7: Arnold-Chiari Type I

notes

retardation. Congenital musculoskeletal, cardiac, and GU disorders also are frequently found; less commonly seen are dental disorders, cleft lip/palate, and disorders of the GI tract, lungs, and skin.

Aim treatment at correcting the associated anomalies, if possible. Risk of serious neurologic sequela is highest with abnormalities at the occipito-C1 junction.

LISSENCEPHALY (AGYRIA)

A brain without cerebral convolutions and a poorly formed sylvian fissure characterizes lissencephaly. It is also usually described as having a smooth cerebral surface with thickened cortical mantle. Luckily, it is rare. Infants who survive to delivery have FTT, microcephaly, marked developmental delay, and severe seizure disorders. They may be blind. ~ 15% occurs in association with Miller-Dieker syndrome (due to deletions of chromosome 17) and presents with prominent forehead, bitemporal "hollowing," anteverted nostrils, prominent upper lip, and micrognathia. CT/MRI will show a "smooth brain" without sulci. (See Figure 11-8.)

SCHIZENCEPHALY

Schizencephaly is the occurrence of unilateral or bilateral clefts within the cerebral hemispheres. CT/MRI is diagnostic and shows the clefts. Infants with bilateral clefts usually have severe seizure disorders, microcephaly, severe mental retardation, and spastic quadriparesis.

PORENCEPHALY

Porencephaly refers to the presence of cysts or cavities within the brain. These may occur due to developmental defects or may be acquired, such as with infarction. "True porencephalic cysts" are located in the sylvian fissure region and communicate with the subarachnoid space, the ventricular system, or both. Infants may have mental retardation, spastic quadriparesis, blindness, and seizures; but they also may be asymptomatic.

"Pseudo-porencephalic" cysts develop during the perinatal or postnatal period and are due to infarction or hemorrhage of the arterial or venous circulation. The cysts are unilateral and usually do not communicate with the ventricular system. They are not associated with other malformations in the CNS. Infants present with hemiparesis and focal seizures during the 1st year of life.

HOLOPROSENCEPHALY

Holoprosencephaly refers to a disorder in the development of the brain itself due to a defective cleavage of the prosencephalon. (Prosencephalon is the anterior primitive cerebral vesicle and the most rostral of the 3 primary brain vesicles of the embryonic neural tube; it subdivides to form the diencephalon and telencephalon.) There are 3 types of holoprosencephaly: 1) alobar, 2) semi-lobar, and 3) lobar. Each is based on the degree of abnormality that occurs in the cleavage process. With holoprosencephaly, facial anomalies are common, particularly cyclopia (one eye), cebocephaly (malformation of the head in which the features are suggestive of a monkey, with a defective or absent nose and close-set eyes), and premaxillary agenesis.

The most severe form is alobar holoprosencephaly, which is associated with having only 1 ventricle, an absent falx, and fused basal ganglia. Most infants die within the first few months.

AGENESIS OF THE CORPUS CALLOSUM

Agenesis of the corpus callosum occurs in a wide variety of disorders, with similar severity variations. Some are asymptomatic and have normal intelligence, while others have severe mental retardation. Isolated agenesis is usually asymptomatic. MRI will show widely separated frontal horns with the 3rd ventricle very high between the lateral ventricles. (See Figure 11-9 showing absence of the corpus callosum in close-up view and Figure 11-10 showing normal corpus callosum.) Absence of the corpus callosum can be inherited as an X-linked recessive trait or an AD trait. It is also associated

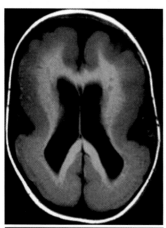

Figure 11-8: Lissencephaly

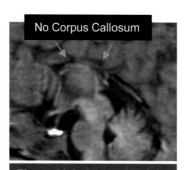

No Corpus Callosum

Figure 11-9: Agenesis of the Corpus Callosum

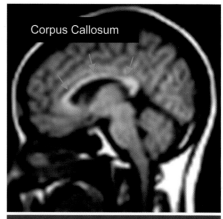

Corpus Callosum

Figure 11-10: Normal MRI

notes

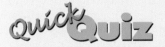

Infantile spasms?

with trisomy 8, trisomy 18, and Aicardi syndrome (a disorder of girls only). Recently, maternal cocaine use has been linked to agenesis of the corpus callosum. Diagnosis is possible from about 20-weeks gestation by ultrasound.

CEREBRAL PALSY

DEFINITIONS

Motor deficits

First, some definitions:

Static encephalopathy refers to "a state of cerebral dysfunction after an insult of limited duration." (Hmm … for me that could happen after taking a Board exam.) The key word is "static," which means the lesion does not progress and may even improve with time.

The following terms are used to describe various abnormalities that develop after a brain insult:
• "Cerebral palsy": involvement of motor areas of the brain.
• "Convulsions": seizures due to cortical lesions.
• "Speech disturbances": may occur due to diffuse cerebral involvement or a focal lesion in the speech area.
• "Behavioral and learning disabilities:" while commonly used, they are not well defined in regard to anatomic injury locations.

So back to cerebral palsy (CP). CP refers to a group of disorders that occur due to a CNS insult during early development that results in chronic, non-progressive afflictions of movement, posture, and tone. The insult may occur before birth, during birth, or shortly after delivery. CP refers only to motor deficits but is frequently associated with seizures, mental retardation, and learning disabilities.

The prevalence of CP is estimated to be ~ 1–2/1,000.

There are 4 types of CP:
• Spastic (70%)
• Dyskinetic (15%) *(athetoxic) – early HIE*
• Ataxic (5%)
• Mixed (10%)

ETIOLOGY

The Bottom Line

The bottom line is: Know that a diverse number of factors are likely involved in CP. None of the factors below, either alone or in combination, have been shown to account for more than a fraction of the total number of cases of children with CP.

Asphyxia

Most once believed that asphyxia during labor and delivery was a major cause of CP, but most now believe asphyxia is not a major cause. Birth asphyxia likely causes only ~ 10–20% of the CP cases. A tight nuchal cord is the only factor associated with birth asphyxia that has a high clinical correlation with development of CP.

Low Birth Weight

There is an increased risk of CP in infants with low birth weight, but the correlation is not linear or absolute. ~ 10% of infants weighing < 1,500 grams develop CP. But, conversely, of all those born with CP, only 10–28% weigh < 1,500 grams at birth. However, a large proportion of children with spastic diplegia (a type of CP that includes bilateral spasticity, with the lower extremities more severely affected) have low birth weight.

Congenital Malformations

The presence of congenital malformations increases the risk of CP. It is known that 22% of children with CP have a major, non-cerebral malformation. Plus, having a congenital malformation increases the risk of perinatal asphyxia, a known risk factor for CP.

Infection

Most believe that infection accounts for ~ 15% of total spastic CP cases in children with normal birth weight. Infection generally results in a much higher incidence of spastic quadriplegia than the diplegic or hemiplegic subtypes (hemiplegia with increased tone in the antigravity muscles of the affected side).

Inflammatory Mediators

Various inflammatory factors are elevated in children with CP. These include IL-1, IL-8, IL-9, TNF-α, and various interferons. A current theory suggests that inflammatory pathways are triggered by an infection—and that the resulting increased inflammatory mediators then either inhibit normal brain development by disrupting myelin or interfere with cell migration. Also, coagulation factors may play a role, with increased risk of a thrombotic phenomenon resulting in damage to the developing brain.

notes

SPASTIC CP

Spastic CP results in upper motor neuron signs, including weakness, hypertonicity with contractures, and hyperreflexia with clonus. [Know]: Since spastic CP involves upper motor neuron signs, abnormal reflexes, such as extensor plantar response, are commonly seen in these children. The upper motor neuron effects of spastic CP can manifest as hemiplegia, quadriplegia, or spastic diplegia (legs with more spasticity than the arms).

DYSKINETIC CP

Dyskinetic CP refers to impaired, willful, yet uncontrolled and purposeless movements that disappear during sleep. The abnormal pathology is in the basal ganglia. The most common type of movement is choreoathetoid. Chorea is the rapid, jerky motion of proximal muscle groups of the arms, legs, and face, while athetosis refers to slow, irregular writhing movements of the arms, legs, face, neck, and torso. The movements become much more exaggerated with emotion, or by intentionally trying to control the movements. Generally, these children have truncal twisting, facial grimacing, and extreme rigidity of their arms and legs, all due to the continual, simultaneous contraction of the agonist and antagonist muscle groups.

ATAXIC CP

Ataxic CP occurs when there is damage to the cerebellum and its pathways. It results in dysfunction of coordination and gait. It is a "static" lesion and does not worsen. These children have a wide-based gait. They cannot perform finger-to-nose pointing well. This type is rare and is a diagnosis of exclusion. It is not associated with neurologic or functional decline, familial ataxia, foot deformities, or sensory deficits; if these do occur, another diagnosis is more likely.

MIXED FORMS

Mixed forms of CP occur most commonly with a combination of spasticity and choreoathetosis. Additionally, athetosis and ataxia may occur.

SEIZURES AND MENTAL RETARDATION

Seizures occur in ~ 25–40% of children with CP. Children with hemiparesis most commonly have seizures, while those with the dyskinetic form have < 10% incidence of seizures. Most seizures begin between ages 2 and 6 years.

Mental retardation occurs within a wide range, 25–75%, depending on which study you read. It is most common in mixed CP and least common in the dyskinetic and ataxic types. It is important to anticipate visual, hearing, and speech disorders in these children.

DIAGNOSIS OF CP

Diagnosis depends on clinical findings. The key: Serial examinations showing a static (non-progressive) disorder. If progression is occurring, you must consider a progressive encephalopathy, especially for metabolic disorders. Ultrasound of the newborn and MRI of older children are helpful in delineating CNS involvement. EEG will help confirm clinically suspected seizures but will not differentiate the etiology.

TREATMENT OF CP

Rehabilitation with physical and occupational therapy is the cornerstone of treatment. Proper stretching and positioning to reduce contractures and assistance with improving gait are paramount. You can control seizures with a variety of agents (see the Seizure Disorders topic later in this section). Spasticity may be improved with diazepam, dantrolene sodium, or baclofen. Botulinum toxin has been used in areas of local spasticity to inhibit release of acetylcholine from motor nerve terminals. Intrathecal baclofen, using a pump, recently has been successful. Surgery with selective dorsal rhizotomy—in which abnormal, afferent dorsal rootlets of L2 to S2 are cut—has been shown to be effective in children with lower extremity spasticity but normal upper extremity function.

CEREBROVASCULAR DISEASES
OVERVIEW

The incidence of stroke in children is increasing and has gone from 2.5/100,000 to 10.7/100,000 in recent series. 45% are ischemic in character. About 1/3 of the ischemic strokes occur in neonates. 75% of strokes are arterial, and 25% are sinovenous thrombosis. Hemorrhagic stroke occurs as frequently as ischemic stroke; hemorrhagic strokes can occur from bleeding into ischemic strokes or from rupture of intracranial arteries. Strokes in children are almost always due to congenital or genetic factors—and not to atherosclerosis, which is the most common cause in adults.

Strokes *in utero* present as early-onset hand dominance or hemiplegic CP.
Perinatal strokes present with focal neonatal seizures; the focal neurologic deficits do not show up for weeks to months.
In children < 2 years of age, a large majority of strokes present with seizures and hemiparesis.
Older children present with an acute focal neurologic deficit, with or without seizures. Fever and mental status changes are common in pediatric strokes.

Acute hemiplegia may be due to stroke, but 3 other diagnoses should be considered in children:
  1) Transient postictal hemiparesis (Todd paralysis) lasts usually 24–48 hours but may last up to 1 week and has

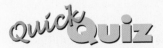

EEG activity consistent with seizures. It is a neuronal exhaustion phenomenon. MRI never shows an acute infarction.

2) Complicated migraine can be preceded by a severe headache, with focal deficits lasting hours—even up to 1 week. Family history is usually positive for hemiplegic migraine. MRI is negative for infarction.

3) Alternating hemiplegia is a rare disorder, generally beginning in children < 2 years of age. The hemiplegia lasts for minutes to hours, with weakness alternating between sides. Seizures are common, but do not occur during the period of weakness. Most children have progressive neurologic or developmental deterioration. The etiology is unknown.

MAJOR CAUSES OF ISCHEMIC STROKES IN CHILDREN

Cardiac Disorders

Congenital heart disease complications cause ~ 25% of pediatric strokes. Most are due to embolic phenomena from the heart or shunted through the heart. Suspect embolic disease if multiple ("showering") infarcts are found on MRI/CT.

Emboli from endocarditis may be infectious or noninfectious. ~ 50% of strokes in children occur within 3 days of catheterization or surgery. Strokes occur in ~ 10% of children who undergo the Fontan procedure and in 5% with valve-replacement surgery without anticoagulation. Tetralogy of Fallot and transposition of the great vessels also predispose to stroke.

Prothrombotic Disorders

About 1/3 of children with ischemic stroke have an abnormality in prothrombotic factors, the most frequent being an acquired antiphospholipid antibody, especially anticardiolipin antibody or lupus anticoagulant. Also, acquired deficiencies can occur due to oral contraceptives, nephrotic syndrome, and liver disease.

Activated protein C resistance (Factor V Leiden) is the most common inheritable cause of venous thrombosis; it can cause arterial thrombosis in older children as well. Activated protein C resistance can cause strokes and hemiplegic CP in neonates. For the hereditary deficiencies, activated protein C resistance is more common than deficiencies of protein C, protein S, or antithrombin. Any of these deficiencies can also result in ischemic stroke.

Sickle-cell Disease

Sickle-cell disease is responsible for ~ 10% of pediatric strokes, which include ischemic strokes, hemorrhagic strokes, or transient ischemic attacks (TIAs). In infants and younger children, ischemic stroke is more likely, while hemorrhagic stroke is more common in adults. Genotype SS has the highest incidence of stroke among the sickle hemoglobinopathies.

Children ages 2–5 have the highest incidence. It is rare to have a stroke in a child < 2 years of age. Higher concentrations of hemoglobin F do not lower the risk of stroke.
~ 20% of children with sickle-cell disease will have MRI/CT evidence of stroke, but no symptoms. Ischemic strokes are rarely fatal, but hemorrhagic strokes have a mortality rate of > 25%. Recurrence of strokes is very common within the first 3 years. You can prevent recurrences with transfusion protocols. Use transcranial Doppler ultrasound to predict which children with sickle-cell disease are at increased risk: mean blood flow > 200 cm/second in either the internal carotid or middle cerebral artery.

Moyamoya disease is a chronic, occlusive, cerebrovascular disease that is associated with sickle-cell disease, as well as neurofibromatosis Type 1, trisomy 21, and cranial irradiation. Moyamoya is a Japanese term meaning "puff of smoke." This refers to extensive collateral vessels resulting from prior occlusions of arteries around the circle of Willis, as seen on cerebral angiography. (See Figure 11-11.)

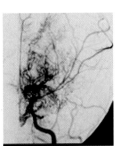

Figure 11-11: Moyamoya

Cervicocephalic Arterial Dissection

Dissections of the cervicocephalic arterial system make up a good percentage of causes of stroke in children and adolescents. The most common arteries affected are the internal carotid arteries. In children, look for focal cerebral symptoms with ipsilateral headache, neck, or eye pain. With internal carotid artery dissection, Horner syndrome, and transient monocular blindness are more commonly seen in adults than children.

Dissections of the internal carotid or vertebral arteries are best diagnosed with cerebral angiography. Magnetic resonance angiography (MRA) can be useful for cervicocephalic arterial dissection. Treatment is controversial. Some recommend

notes

anticoagulation, but, for intracranial vessel dissections, anticoagulation is contraindicated because of the increased risk of subarachnoid hemorrhage.

CNS Vasculitis

Bacterial meningitis is the most common cause of CNS vasculitis. Infarction is found in ~ 25% of children with bacterial meningitis and is typically a venous infarct secondary to retrograde thrombophlebitis. Tuberculosis may cause arterial infarcts.

Recently, chickenpox has been increasingly reported as being associated with incidence of stroke. The cases occurred in children < 10 years of age; the infarcts were in the basal ganglia or internal capsule. Most occurred within 9 months of the chickenpox rash. Some retrospective studies indicate that 17% of children with stroke had an episode of chickenpox in the previous 6 months. It appears that the varicella issue relates to post-infectious vasculopathy.

CNS lupus has a 6% incidence of CNS vasculitis in adults, but < 2% in children. Inflammatory bowel disease has about a 3% risk of CNS vasculitis in children.

Takayasu arteritis is rare in the U.S., but in affected Asian females, 5–10% develop strokes. Immunosuppression is the treatment of choice.

Cocaine and "diet pill" use has been associated with an increased risk of vasculopathy and vasospasm.

Metabolic Etiologies

Metabolic causes of stroke are rare in children but can be due to Fabry disease and homocystinuria, both of which can cause vascular occlusion. Fabry disease causes deficiency of α-galactosidase, which causes accumulation of ceramide trihexoside in vascular endothelium that in turn leads to arterial narrowing, ischemia, and eventual infarction. Homocystinuria causes injury to vascular endothelium, leading to thrombus formation. Measure serum homocystine levels in all children with ischemic stroke since recent data have shown that homocystine levels are elevated due to a large variety of etiologies, both genetic and environmental, including vitamin deficiencies, renal disease, drugs such as phenytoin and theophylline, cigarettes, and hypothyroidism. However, the significance of elevated homocystine levels has become controversial.

MELAS is a syndrome of mitochondrial myopathy, encephalopathy, lactic acidosis, and stroke-like episodes that usually presents in children ages 5–15 years. More on these can be found in the Metabolic Disorders section.

NEONATAL CEREBRAL INFARCTION

Neonatal cerebral infarction is considered separately because of the increased prevalence compared to older children. Most neonatal cerebral infarctions occur in full-term infants, but some preterm infants also can be affected. It is estimated to occur in 1/4,000 infants.

Most neonatal cerebral infarctions are embolic and occur in the distribution of the left middle cerebral artery. Many believe that the placenta may be the source for some of these emboli. Other causes include hypoxic-ischemic encephalopathy (see next), pro-thrombotic conditions (see above), and acute, severe hypertension.

Hypoxic-ischemic encephalopathy (HIE) is thought by some to cause a good percentage of cerebral accidents in neonates. Brain injury can occur due to hypoxia, ischemia, asphyxia, and acidosis. Preterm infants show weakness of the lower extremities due to periventricular leukomalacia. Full-term infants have quadriparesis due to parasagittal brain involvement. HIE is usually diffuse but, on occasion, can be focal.

The most common presentation for infants with neonatal cerebral infarction is focal seizures within the first 3–4 days of life.

MRI is the best diagnostic tool for strokes in neonates. Early on, there may be only subtle changes, but over time the infarct becomes clearer on MRI. Many recommend using diffusion-weighted imaging, which will pick up the lesion earlier and can help "date" the stroke.

Aim management at treating any confounding, underlying causes, and treat seizures with anticonvulsants. Usually, you can stop the anti-seizure medications in ~ 6 months because these infants rarely go on to have persistent seizure disorders.

HEMORRHAGIC STROKE

Hemorrhagic stroke in children is as common as ischemic stroke. Bleeding of normal vessels occurs due to head trauma or coagulopathies; and abnormal vessels bleed because of vascular malformations or aneurysms. Bleeding can be subarachnoid, intraparenchymal, or both.

Children with intraparenchymal bleeding present with headache, focal neurologic findings, seizures, and mental status changes. Large bleeds usually cause coma. Neonates have signs of increased intracranial pressure. Subarachnoid hemorrhage presents with "the worst headache of my life," followed by findings of meningeal irritation and increased intracranial pressure.

You can see acute bleeds easily on a non-contrast CT scan. Head trauma is the most common cause of intracranial bleeding and is very common in the "shaken baby" syndrome. Coagulopathies are the next most common cause of bleeding; however, trauma is usually a precipitating event although the trauma can be very minor.

Vascular malformations may be arteriovenous, cavernous, venous angiomas, or capillary telangiectasias. Arteriovenous malformations (AVMs) are abnormal collections of arteries and veins without the normal intervening capillary bed. Smaller AVMs appear with focal seizures, while those with large AVMs present with headache, focal neurologic findings, intracranial bruit, and seizures. AVMs require embolization or surgical removal.

Cavernous malformations are collections of thin-walled vessels with only a single layer of endothelium—and nothing else. Recurrent bleeding is common, but the lesions are rarely life-threatening. Enhanced MRI can detect these fairly easily.

Venous angiomas are the most common vascular malformation. Most children with these are asymptomatic, but some may

notes

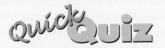
present with seizures. CT/MRI will show the lesions. Even when symptomatic, venous angiomas rarely require surgery, and, in fact, surgery may increase the severity and frequency of symptoms.

Saccular aneurysms are usually asymptomatic and less common than AVMs. They are associated with coarctation of the aorta, polycystic kidneys, Ehlers-Danlos syndrome, and Marfan syndrome. Usually, the aneurysms come off of the internal carotid artery or anterior cerebral artery. These aneurysms, although usually asymptomatic, may cause acute subarachnoid hemorrhage, which results in the "worst headache of my life" scenario described above. If subarachnoid hemorrhage occurs, surgery is the treatment of choice.

CEREBRAL VEIN THROMBOSIS

Cerebral vein thrombosis is an important cause of stroke in infants and children. Its incidence is estimated to be 0.67 cases/100,000 children a year. Neonates are most commonly affected. Symptoms depend on which vessel is occluded.

Superior sagittal sinus thrombosis leads to obstruction to CSF absorption and causes increased intracranial pressure. The cortical veins from the superior surface of each cerebral hemisphere drain into the superior sagittal sinus. Patients present with headache, papilledema, nausea, vomiting, and 6th cranial nerve palsy.

Right lateral sinus (the superior sagittal sinus empties into the right lateral sinus) thrombosis was very common with otitis media and mastoiditis in the pre-antibiotic era. Cranial nerves were frequently affected. It is still one of the causes of pseudotumor cerebri, characterized by papilledema and 6th nerve palsy, which are due to the increased intracranial pressure.

Cavernous sinuses drain blood from the orbits, middle cerebral veins, and the anterior undersurface of the brain; the cavernous sinuses then drain into the internal jugular veins via the petrosal sinuses. Thrombosis of the cavernous sinuses results in proptosis, chemosis, and uni- or bilateral ophthalmoplegia. Thrombosis of the cavernous sinuses occurs most commonly due to infection of the paranasal sinuses, face, nose, or mouth.

In neonates with any of these cerebral venous thromboses, seizures are the most common clinical presentation. For older children, headache and vomiting are most common.

Risk factors for cerebral venous thrombosis usually include pro-thrombotic conditions and especially dehydration. Infection is also a common predisposing factor.

CT scan may be initially normal in 40%. Contrast is usually required, and "the empty delta sign" occurs after contrast is injected and presents as a filling defect of the superior sagittal sinus. MRI with magnetic resonance venogram (MRV) is the best method of diagnosis.

Management is controversial. In adults, good data exist that suggest anticoagulation is beneficial even in hemorrhagic lesions. Data in children are minimal but appear to parallel the adult data. In one study, death and high morbidity occurred in ~ 1/3 of infants and children.

INJURY / TRAUMA TO THE CENTRAL AND PERIPHERAL NERVOUS SYSTEMS

OCCURRENCE

Accidents account for 40% of all pediatric deaths, making them the leading cause of pediatric mortality overall. Head injury makes up a good proportion of these accidents. The incidence of head trauma in children age 0–19 years is 2/1,000, with 1/10,000 of those dying from their head trauma. Boys have an incidence 2x that of girls. In older children, motor vehicle accidents and sports-related injuries are the leading causes of head injury. In younger children, falls rank as the leading cause of head injury.

SCALP INJURIES

Lacerations

Scalp lacerations lead to marked and alarming bleeding because of the rich anastomotic blood supply of the scalp, as well as the limited ability of the vessels in the dense connective tissue layer to contract/retract. Large lacerations heal very well, and infection is rare. Primary closure is best, but if conditions prevent immediate intervention, you can delay it for 8–12 hours without increasing the risk of infection.

Hematomas

Hematomas of the scalp are common in children, but they are usually not very large and absorb within 2–3 days. If a galeal laceration occurs, it may permit bleeding from above to permeate the subgaleal connective tissue layer and results in a quick-forming, extensive swelling that is of enormous size.

notes

The swelling occurs because there is no limiting membrane to prevent its spread. Cephalohematomas occur in newborns and some older children; these are discussed in The Fetus & Newborn section.

Skull Fractures

Skull fractures vary in size, shape, and location. They can occur as isolated events but, unfortunately, are more commonly associated with underlying cerebral injury. More on skull fractures in the Emergency Pediatric Care section.

More than 80% of skull fractures are simple linear or diastatic fractures; the parietal area is the most common location. Diastatic fractures usually involve the lambdoid suture, with a spread > 1.5 mm considered abnormal.

Children < 1 year have craniums that are not well calcified; thus bones may be displaced inward without an actual break and produce what is known as a "ping-pong" or "pond" fracture.

Bilateral orbital ecchymoses ("raccoon eyes" or black eyes) may indicate a fracture at the base of the skull. Such a fracture also might be indicated by posterior auricular ecchymoses ("Battle sign") and tympanic membrane discoloration if the petrous bone of the middle fossa is involved. Otorrhea and rhinorrhea can indicate a basilar skull fracture. Air collected in the meningeal spaces (aerocele) or the ventricular system (pneumoencephalocele) implies fractures through the paranasal sinuses.

In all children < 3 years of age, skull x-rays are usually done for all but trivial head injury. If you suspect an underlying intracranial lesion, you generally would not do plain films of the skull. Instead, use CT scan with bone windows.

Suspect underlying lesions in any of the following:
- Depressed or comminuted skull fracture
- Loss of consciousness lasting at least 5 minutes
- Altered mental status or irritability
- Bulging fontanelle
- Focal neurologic signs or deteriorating neurologic condition
- Vomiting at least 5 times or for more than 6 hours
- Nonimpact seizures
- In children < 6 months of age

Use skeletal surveys and cervical spinal films in trauma situations—or if you suspect abuse.

Children who have partially recovered by the time they make it to the ER usually have few signs on examination. Most of these patients can be managed at home if observed 6–8 hours after injury, which is the time interval for most acute intracranial bleeds to develop.

Simple linear fractures do not require specific therapy, and the child's normal activities should not be restricted. Repeat skull x-ray in 3 months to show union. Most fractures heal within 6–12 months. A late complication of linear fracture is a leptomeningeal cyst, which results from dural laceration, especially in the parietal area. The cyst can result in projection of the arachnoid membrane into the fracture site, with brain herniation causing bone erosion of the overlying skull over months or years. This complication is suggested by late onset of focal seizures, focal neurologic signs, and an occasional visible and palpable skull deformity. Skull x-rays are diagnostic, showing bony erosion over a prior fracture site. Nearly 50% occur in children < 1 year of age, with 90% of the total accounted for in the "under age 3" group.

"Ping-pong" or pond fractures do not usually require surgical elevation unless they are depressed > 0.5 cm. Observe most pond fractures regularly for 3 months.

Basilar skull fractures that result in otorrhea or rhinorrhea should be observed in the hospital. Plugging or irrigating the nose or ear is contraindicated. Antibiotics are not recommended prophylactically. CSF will usually stop draining within 72 hours. If it hasn't, closed system, spinal fluid drainage from the lumbar subarachnoid space for an additional 72 hours may be helpful. If this fails, perform surgery. Suppress coughing and sneezing.

PARENCHYMAL INJURIES

Cerebral Contusion

Cerebral contusions are ecchymoses of the brain and are usually located on the surface. Contusions can result in focal neurologic findings. Contusions can occur directly under the blunt trauma or could be distant from the site of impact, as in an acceleration-deceleration injury. For example, a blow to the occiput could cause frontal or temporal lobe injury, depending on the direction of the force.

Diffuse Axonal Injury

Diffuse axonal injury is seen most commonly with acceleration-deceleration injuries from motor vehicle accidents. The gray matter and white matter have different densities, so force will result in different acceleration and deceleration for each and in shearing of the white matter, usually at the gray-white matter junction. In the absence of brain contusion, axonal injury is frequently responsible for prolonged alteration in alertness level and cognitive function.

Epidural Hematoma

Epidural hematoma is bleeding that occurs between the skull and the dura. (See Figure 11-12.) It most commonly occurs with: 1) a temporal bone fracture, which causes a tear of the middle meningeal artery; or 2) more commonly in children, from a tear in the bridging veins or dural sinuses. Untreated, mortality is ~ 100%.

The scenario is classic. Look for a child on the Board exam who is unconscious by trauma, regains consciousness over several hours, and then worsens. Epidural hematomas of arterial origin can grow rapidly—and acutely raise intracranial pressure, which results in hypertension, bradycardia, and a progressive decline in mental status. Focal seizures may occur. Because the pressure increase is so rapid—and is frequently asymmetric in character—the cerebral contents may be shifted away from the lesion, resulting in herniation of the tip of the temporal lobe and compression of the midbrain.

notes

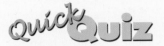

Quick Quiz

1) In what area of the skull does a fracture most commonly occur in children?

2) What type of fracture is indicated by bilateral "raccoon eyes"?

3) What type of fracture is indicated by otorrhea and rhinorrhea?

4) When would you do a CT scan with bone windows, instead of plain skull x-rays, in a child < 3 years with suspected skull fracture?

5) How are most uncomplicated linear skull fractures managed?

6) When do pond fractures of the skull require surgical elevation?

7) Which type of basilar skull fractures requires observation in the hospital?

8) Under what conditions are you most likely to see diffuse axonal injury?

9) Describe an epidural hematoma.

10) What is the classic presentation for a child with epidural hematoma?

11) How does "early herniation" present in a child with epidural hematoma?

12) What are some of the more common causes of spinal injury?

Early herniation is characterized by a dilated pupil on the side of the hematoma progressing to a complete 3rd nerve palsy and a contralateral hemiplegia (opposite to the lesion). In late stages, both pupils become fixed and dilated, respiration is slow and irregular, and hypotension and tachycardia develop.

Subdural Hematoma

Subdural hematomas are common in children < 1 year. (See Figure 11-13.) Acute presentation may be within 3 days of the trauma; subacute, from 3 days to nearly 3 weeks later; or chronic, > 3 weeks afterward. Acute lesions are usually arterial and require emergent care. The "shaken-baby" syndrome, as well as bacterial meningitis, is responsible for some chronic subdural lesions.

Subdural paracentesis is diagnostic and therapeutic. Daily removal of ~ 10 mL of fluid decreases the intracranial pressure, while also decreasing the size of the hematoma. Do not remove > 20 mL of fluid, because this will likely increase re-accumulation. Recovery is generally excellent if no underlying, parenchymal damage exists.

SPINAL CORD INJURY

Spinal injuries are somewhat common in children. The most common etiologies are motor vehicle accidents, falls, and swimming pool injuries (diving). In neonates, trauma during delivery is the most common etiology.

Younger children, age < 3 years, have an increased proportion of cervical and upper thoracic spine injuries, as well as a higher frequency of spinal cord injury without radiographic abnormalities. This type of lesion has a poorer prognosis.

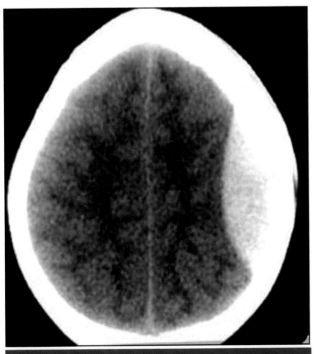

Figure 11-12: Epidural Hematoma

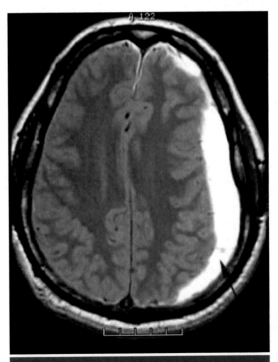

Figure 11-13: Subdural Hematoma

notes

Spinal cord injury ranges from "whiplash"—in which the spine is hyperextended or over-flexed with musculoskeletal symptoms—to complex severing or infarction of the cord.

In newborns, use the Gallant response to help determine the extent of damage in the thoracic cord. In this reflex, scratch the paraspinal region to elicit incurvation of the spine toward the side of the stimulus; with injury, the reflex is absent at that level.

"Spinal shock" is a period of flaccidity and areflexia and can occur following an acute injury. After 2 weeks, it progresses to varying degrees of spasticity and hyperreflexia. Use spinal MRI to generally delineate the problem.

Give children with acute spinal cord injury IV methylprednisolone, which has been to shown to enhance motor and sensory recovery in adult studies. Never manipulate cervical spine injuries to reduce a fracture.

COMMON PERIPHERAL NERVE INJURIES

Birth Trauma

Birth trauma is the most common cause of peripheral nerve injury. The brachial plexus has points of fixation to the 1st rib medially and the coracoid process of the scapula laterally. Forced abduction of the arm stretches the nerves under and against the coracoid and can result in stretching, avulsing, or compressing the lower plexus. Lateral deviation of the head and depression of the shoulder will result in similar constriction to the upper plexus. Injuries of this type can occur with breech or cephalic deliveries.

Risk factors include macrosomia, use of forceps, shoulder dystocia, and gestational diabetes. ~ 50% are due to shoulder dystocia.

Erb-Duchenne Type Injuries (Upper Plexus Root)

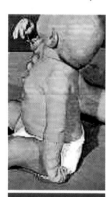

Figure 11-14: Erb Palsy

Upper plexus root injuries are the most common peripheral nerve injuries. The infant presents with a sagging shoulder, an arm that hangs limp in internal rotation, and a pronated wrist. (See Figure 11-14.) Symptoms are due to paralysis of the spinate, deltoid, biceps, brachioradialis, and extensor carpi radialis muscles. The biceps tendon reflex is absent, but the triceps reflex is present. Sensory examination is normal. Treatment involves placing the arm in abduction and external rotation. > 90% will have a full recovery within 3 months. Surgery can attempted in those who don't improve.

Klumpke-Dejerine Type Injuries (Lower Plexus Root)

Lower plexus root injuries (C8–T1) show more sensory (ulnar side of the hand) and vasomotor involvement, with paralysis of the flexors and extensors of the forearm and intrinsic muscles of the hand. If the 1st thoracic root is involved, Horner syndrome and cervical sympathetic damage is likely. Treat by splinting the forearm and wrist in a neutral position. Most recover in 3–6 months but don't do as well as those with upper plexus root injury. Surgery with microvascular techniques may be beneficial.

Serratus Anterior Palsy

Serratus anterior palsy is due to involvement of the long thoracic nerve and is usually caused by pressure on the shoulder or excessive throwing activity with the arms elevated. As such, this is most common in boys who pitch baseballs, lift weights, or carry heavy loads. Use of an arm sling during the 1st week will alleviate discomfort. Treat with range-of-motion exercises, followed by active shoulder-strengthening exercises.

Sciatic Nerve Injury

Sciatic nerve injury is most commonly iatrogenic with intramuscular injections. IM injections during infancy are contraindicated in the intragluteal area and should be done with extreme caution in older children. Complete sciatic paralysis produces total foot paralysis and loss of leg flexion. It also results in flail footdrop, absence of ankle jerk reflex, and sensory loss of the leg below the knee, except for the medial portion. Consider surgery in infants, but note that high lesions rarely fully recover.

SEIZURE DISORDERS

OCCURRENCE

Seizures occur before age 20 years in ~ 5% of middle-socioeconomic-class populations; the incidence in low-socioeconomic groups is twice as high. Seizures occur most frequently in infants and the elderly. The incidence is ~ 9/10,000 in the 1st year of life; ~ 6/10,000 for ages 1–5; ~ 5/10,000 for ages 5–9; and ~ 4/10,000 for ages 10–14.

PRIMARY GENERALIZED SEIZURES

Mechanism / Characteristics

Generalized seizures involve both cerebral hemispheres from the beginning of the seizure. Generalized seizures make up 60% of all seizures in childhood, making them the most common type seen.

Certain characteristics are classic for generalized seizures:
• Abrupt onset.
• Loss or alteration of consciousness.
• Variable bilateral symmetric motor activity associated with changes in muscle tone.
• No warning of the attack; no aura.
• EEG shows epileptiform activity that is bilateral and synchronous.

notes

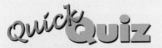
Tonic-Clonic Seizures (Grand Mal Seizure)

Tonic-clonic seizures are the classic form of generalized-onset seizures. Note, however: The combined tonic-clonic event is rare in infancy but not uncommon in early childhood—due to the commonality of simple febrile seizures, which are generalized tonic-clonic in nature. Besides febrile seizures, most seizures in the younger age groups are either tonic or clonic in character.

The "tonic" phase occurs first, with loss of consciousness simultaneous with marked, sustained contractions of the entire musculature. With these movements, the eyes deviate conjugately upward. During this phase, there is pupillary dilation, salivation, diaphoreses, and increased blood pressure. Urinary incontinence is common. The tonic phase lasts 10–20 seconds; this is followed by the "clonic" phase, which is a series of relaxations of all muscle groups and results in interruption of the sustained, tonic muscular spasm. The clonic phase lasts 30 seconds.

After the seizure in the postictal period, the child slowly regains full consciousness and is typically confused and sleepy from a few minutes to several hours. Once fully awake, he/she may complain of headache and muscle aches, but otherwise cannot remember the seizure event.

Myoclonic Seizures

Assoc c Metabolic d/o

Myoclonic seizures are classically defined by:
- short duration;
- rapid, bilateral, symmetric muscle contractions;
- isolated or repetitive jerks; and
- likelihood of the patient falling (if severe).

Myoclonic seizures can be isolated or may occur with absence attacks or tonic-clonic attacks. With brief attacks, consciousness may be maintained; prolonged attacks typically impact consciousness more.

Myoclonic seizures are best treated with valproate or other broad-spectrum anticonvulsants. Often, myoclonic seizures are associated with other seizure types and with progressive neurodegenerative genetic diseases.

Juvenile Myoclonic Epilepsy (Janz Syndrome)

Juvenile myoclonic epilepsy is a subtype of idiopathic generalized epilepsy. It is also known as "impulsive petit mal." It is characterized by:
- morning myoclonic jerks,
- +/– history of absence seizures,
- generalized tonic-clonic seizures occurring just after awaking or during sleep,
- normal intelligence,
- family history of similar seizures, and *teenager*
- onset at 8–20 years of age.

AM szs + dropping things

This condition is usually lifelong. Seizures increase with sleep deprivation, stress, or alcohol use. Valproate is the drug of choice. *Good outcome*

Absence Seizures (Petit Mal Seizures)

Absence seizures are classically characterized by:
- episodes of extremely short lapses in awareness,
- amnesia during the episodes,
- short duration (rarely longer than a few seconds— 10 seconds at most),
- abrupt onset and end (frequently in mid-conversation or activity), and
- flickering of the eyelids, staring, or eye rolling.

Complex (atypical) absence seizures may additionally have:
- brief jerks of the eyelids and limbs,
- transient change in postural tone (increase or decrease),
- pupillary dilatation,
- skin-color changes,
- tachycardia, and
- not associated with auras, hallucinations, or postictal abnormalities.

Absence seizures can be confused with complex partial seizures, but the latter often last longer (usually > 30 seconds), have auras, and have slow return to consciousness.

Absence seizures occur generally between the ages of 3 and 12 years, with a peak between 4 and 8 years, and are more common in girls. They can occur many times in a day. Hyperventilation for 3–4 minutes can produce an absence seizure. EEG shows a typical 3/sec generalized spike and wave discharge. Treat with ethosuximide, lamotrigine, or valproate.

if no GTC

There is a multifactorial, familial form known as childhood absence epilepsy. It occurs in children ages 4–12. Those affected have normal intelligence, normal neurologic examination, normal EEG interictally, and no family history of tonic-clonic epilepsy; ~ 90% will eventually become seizure-free. Treat with ethosuximide or valproate.

notes

Atonic or Akinetic Seizures (Epileptic Drop Attacks)

An atonic seizure has the following characteristics:
- Without warning, a sudden and complete loss of tone in the limbs, neck, and trunk muscles.
- Can be brief or longer duration.
- Loss of consciousness.
- Complete awareness returns very quickly after the attack.
- One or more myoclonic jerks may occur immediately before muscle tone is lost.

Atonic seizures are more common in children with static encephalopathies and are frequently difficult to treat.

PARTIAL (FOCAL) SEIZURES

Occurrence   Get imaging

Focal seizures are less common in children than adults but still make up 40–45% of childhood seizures. Children rarely have a definable "focal" lesion responsible for their focal seizure. < 10% of children with focal seizures have brain tumors or AVMs as etiology. Other children may have had strokes or cortical malformations. Finally, those with Sturge-Weber disease—where the hemisphere unilateral to the facial port wine nevus often has angiomatosis—may have contralateral focal seizures.

Simple Partial Seizures

Simple partial seizures can be quite varied in symptoms/signs and can be focal-motor (from the precentral gyrus), focal-adversive (from the mesial frontal lobe), or focal-somatosensory (from the parietal lobe) in character. They usually last 10–20 seconds. Focal motor findings are the most common and include asynchronous clonic or tonic movements that tend to involve the face, neck, and extremities. Aura can occur, as well as chest discomfort or headache. Complex emotional or hallucinatory phenomena are common. The term "simple" means that the patients can still interact with their environment without loss of consciousness. There is no postictal confusion. Simple partial seizures may be followed by Todd paralysis, a transient paralysis of the affected body part lasting for minutes or hours.

Complex Partial Seizures

Complex partial seizures have variable symptoms but usually include alterations in consciousness, unresponsiveness, and automatisms. Automatisms are repetitive, purposeless, undirected, and inappropriate motor activities. Commonly, they include repetitive lip smacking, swallowing, chewing, or fidgeting of the fingers or hands. Prior to the seizure, a typical aura is not uncommon, and children may report a sense of detachment or depersonalization, forced thinking, visual distortions, or hallucinations. Feelings of intense emotion or fear also can occur. Postictally, patients are confused and recover consciousness slowly. During the postictal time period, these children tend to act aggressively or angrily to objects or persons that are in their way; this does not occur as a manifestation of the seizure itself.

Most complex partial seizures are due to abnormalities in the limbic structures; these include the hippocampus, amygdala, and mesial temporal lobe. EEG will frequently show spikes or sharp waves over one or both temporal lobes. However, some foci from the orbitofrontal cortex or occipital lobe can spread into the limbic area and mimic these seizures. The most common structural abnormality in these children is mesial temporal sclerosis.

Treatment of complex partial seizures can be very difficult; seizures are completely controlled in < 1/3. The drugs of choice are carbamazepine, oxcarbazepine, or phenytoin. Some children require temporal lobectomy, especially those who have uncontrolled seizures that arise from the anterior temporal lobe on one side.

INFANTILE SPASMS (WEST SYNDROME)

Infantile spasms are a unique type of seizure disorder occurring in infants and children < 1 year. A majority have spasms at ages 4–8 months. (< 10% present after age 2 years.) The classic "spasm" is the flexor spasm, or "salaam attack Blitz-Krampf." These children have sudden, simultaneous flexion of their head and trunk, with flexion and adduction of their extremities. The spasms typically occur in clusters of diminishing severity. The number of clusters can vary from a few to too-numerous-to-count (> 100). The spasms can be initiated or aggravated by transitions from sleep to wakefulness or by feeding, handling, or emotions.

The EEG is very abnormal in children with infantile spasms and is known as hypsarrhythmia: high-voltage, irregular, slow waves that occur out of synch and randomly over all head regions, and intermixed with spikes and multiple spikes from multiple foci.

Cerebral dysgenesis, genetic and metabolic disorders (PKU, tuberous sclerosis), intrauterine infections, and hypoxic-ischemic brain damage are the most commonly identified etiologies. DPT vaccine was once thought to have some role, but that has now been completely dismissed as causative.

Infantile spasms resolve over time even without specific therapy; but most surviving children, unfortunately, have severe mental retardation and other types of seizure disorders. Mortality is ~ 20%.

Treatment is controversial, and the spasms are refractory to therapy. Hormonal therapy with ACTH is the most common treatment in the U.S. Response usually occurs within 2 weeks of starting therapy and lands at either extreme: complete or nonexistent. An emerging therapy for children with infantile spasms is vigabatrin, which was approved by the FDA in August 2009.

notes

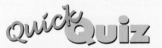

LENNOX-GASTAUT SYNDROME

Lennox-Gastaut syndrome refers to a varied group of symptoms with severe seizures, mental retardation, and a characteristic EEG pattern. The EEG has generalized, bilateral synchronous, sharp-wave and slow-wave complexes, occurring in a repetitive fashion in long runs at ~ 2/second.

The syndrome does not have a specific etiology but can be due to any cause of diffuse encephalopathy, including cerebral malformation, perinatal asphyxia, head injury, anoxic encephalopathy, infection, or postimmunization encephalopathies. ~ 1/3 are idiopathic.

Seizures begin in the first 3 years of life and are refractory to medications. Younger children have atonic, tonic, and atypical absence seizures, while older children have tonic-clonic seizures. Most children have 2 or more different kinds of seizures on a daily basis.

Prognosis is poor, with most children having seizures into adulthood. Drug therapy is empiric at best with valproate, lamotrigine, felbamate, and topiramate available.

POST-TRAUMATIC SEIZURES

Head trauma can result in seizures at any age. The seizures can occur within 1–2 weeks after the injury (early post-traumatic), as a coinciding reaction to the brain trauma, or months to years after the injury (late post-traumatic). The risk of a seizure disorder after a head injury is directly related to the severity of the head injury. Greatest risk is seen with intracerebral hematoma, cerebral contusion, or unconsciousness lasting > 24 hours. Those children with mild head injury and momentary unconsciousness without skull fracture or neurologic deficit have no increased risk of later seizures.

OTHER SEIZURE TYPES

Flickering-Light or Video Game-Induced Seizures

Intermittent or flickering light—especially strobe lights, sunlight through trees, or video games—rarely provokes myoclonic seizures with or without absence or tonic-clonic seizures. Almost always, these begin at ages 8–19 years. Some children can self-induce the attacks by waving their hand in front of their eyes. EEG shows bilateral, synchronous, spike-wave discharges that are irregular in occurrence. This is an uncommon presentation of epilepsy in children.

Treatment usually involves limiting the provoking stimulus; dark glasses are helpful in some children. For drug therapy, valproate is considered the best.

Acquired Epileptic Aphasia (Landau-Kleffner Syndrome)

Acquired epileptic aphasia is likely not a true seizure disorder, but its symptoms justify covering the subject in this section. Healthy children will present with acute or intermittent episodes of losing previously acquired language skills. The aphasia usually begins as a verbal auditory agnosia. EEG findings show slowing and high-voltage seizure activity that may be temporal, bitemporal, or generalized. Anti-seizure drugs have little effect; some tout corticosteroids. About 2/3 of children will have residual language deficit.

Epilepsia Partialis Continua

Epilepsia partialis continua is a syndrome of simple, focal status epilepticus that most commonly occurs in children < age 10. It may be associated with Rasmussen syndrome.

Rasmussen Syndrome

Many believe Rasmussen syndrome to be an immunologic process involving one hemisphere of the brain. ~ 70% have a history of infectious or inflammatory illness themselves or in a family member. Initially, the seizures may be generalized but soon become focal, unremitting, and limited to one part

Table 11-1: Preferred Drugs for Seizure Disorders

Partial and secondary generalized seizures	Carbamazepine, oxcarbazepine, or topiramate
Absence seizures	Ethosuximide, lamotrigine, or valproic acid
Idiopathic generalized tonic-clonic seizures	Valproate, topiramate, or carbamazepine–contraindicated if spike wave pattern on EEG
Complex partial seizures	Carbamazepine, phenytoin, or oxcarbazepine
More than one type of seizure present	Valproate

notes

or side of the body. Eventually, hemiparesis, diminished intelligence, and hemianopia occur. The disease is not fatal but deteriorates to a stable neurologic deficit.

Medical therapy is disappointing—especially antiseizure medications. Corticosteroids and immunologic therapies may be useful, but more studies are needed. A modified hemispherectomy or focal cortical excision can improve symptoms markedly.

Other Seizures

Gelastic seizures occur in children and present as pathologic laughter without an appropriate reason for laughing. They are usually complex-partial in nature and often associated with hypothalamic hamartomas. Cursive epilepsy refers to children with complex partial seizures who present with running as the main symptom! Reflex epilepsy is a seizure disorder that is "set up" by a particular stimulus, such as a pattern, picture, or a light tap/touch.

DRUG THERAPY AND SIDE EFFECTS

Valproate (Valproic Acid)

Use valproate for generalized tonic-clonic, absence, atypical absence, and myoclonic seizures. Many avoid the use of valproate in preschool children because of the risk of severe hepatotoxicity. More common side effects include weight gain, hair loss, and dose-related thrombocytopenia (associated with viral infections). Less common side effects include pancreatitis. Recent reports and data suggest that valproate has an increased risk of teratogenicity versus other antiseizure drugs, as well as an increased risk of having elevated umbilical levels compared to maternal levels. Many recommend avoiding valproic acid in pregnancy if seizures can be controlled by another agent.

Some feel that L-carnitine levels may be decreased, possibly aggravating or initiating these syndromes, and thus some recommend L-carnitine supplementation, especially in children < 2 years of age.

Carbamazepine

Carbamazepine is useful for focal seizures, with or without secondary generalizations. Serious but rare side effects include severe leukopenia and hepatotoxicity during the initial 4 months of therapy. Other side effects include dizziness, drowsiness, diplopia, and SIADH. Avoid erythromycin because it will elevate carbamazepine levels.

Phenytoin

Phenytoin is not commonly used in children due to its zero-order kinetic metabolism. When used, it works best for partial seizures, with and without secondary generalization. It has many side effects, including hirsutism, gum hypertrophy, ataxia, skin rash, Stevens-Johnson syndrome, nystagmus, drowsiness, and blood dyscrasias.

Ethosuximide

Ethosuximide is the drug of choice for absence seizures. Side effects include abdominal pain, skin rash, liver dysfunction, and leukopenia. It is not used for any other seizure types.

Phenobarbital

Phenobarbital is useful for generalized tonic-clonic seizures and partial seizures. It is most commonly used in neonates and infants. Do not use in older children, because many patients have severe behavioral changes or impairment of cognition while on the drug. It is not known whether these changes may persist once the medication is discontinued. Otherwise, its side effect profile is good, and the drug does not require routine laboratory work. It is still used for status epilepticus.

Oxcarbazepine

Oxcarbazepine was recently approved for adjunctive and monotherapy for partial seizures in children aged 4–16 years. Side effects include somnolence, vomiting, ataxia, rash, and nystagmus. Hyponatremia was seen in 2.5% of patients in pre-FDA approval trials.

Lamotrigine

Lamotrigine is approved for partial seizures, generalized seizures of Lennox-Gastaut syndrome, and primary generalized tonic-clonic seizures in children > 2 years. The agent has a "black box" warning for Stevens-Johnson syndrome, with an incidence of 8/1,000 in pediatric patients.

STATUS EPILEPTICUS

Status epilepticus is defined as repeated seizures without regaining consciousness or a seizure prolonged for at least 20 minutes. They may be convulsive (tonic-clonic), nonconvulsive (absence or complex partial), partial (epilepsia partialis continua), or subclinical (electrographic status epilepticus). Underlying disorders, such as sepsis, meningitis, trauma, or encephalopathies, are common. Children seem to tolerate status epilepticus better than adults. Morbidity is most affected by hypoxia, hypotension, and hyperthermia—so you must control these quickly and effectively. The ABCs of airway, breathing, and circulation must be the first priority. Give high-flow oxygen, insert an oral airway, and infuse 10% glucose. Keep total fluid < 1,000 mL/m^2.

Initially, slowly infuse an IV dose of diazepam (0.3–0.5 mg/kg, not to exceed 10 mg) or lorazepam (0.05–0.1 mg/kg, up to 2 mg). A rectal gel formulation of diazepam is now available. Repeat the dose if seizures persist. Also, give fosphenytoin at a dose of 15–20 mg/kg. You can give additional smaller doses, as needed, until clinical seizures are controlled.

Alternatively, phenobarbital may be used. Give as 10–20 mg/kg IV, and repeat if seizures continue. Be sure to monitor vital signs.

If there is still no improvement, a combination of fosphenytoin and phenobarbital and/or general anesthesia may be required. Midazolam has been used in continuous infusion in some instances.

notes

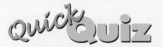

Quick Quiz

1) Why is valproate avoided in young children?
2) Which antibiotic should be avoided with carbamazepine use?
3) Describe the pharmacokinetics of phenytoin.
4) What is the drug of choice for absence seizures?
5) Should you use phenobarbital in older children?
6) Define status epilepticus.
7) Which drugs increase the risk of neural tube defects in infants of pregnant women on these medications?
8) Is it okay for a woman on seizure medications to breastfeed?
9) What are some common etiologies of neonatal seizures?
10) In an infant with a seizure, is lumbar puncture indicated?

COMMON EPILEPSY QUESTIONS

When to Stop Therapy?

Neurologically normal children with idiopathic epilepsy, whose seizures come readily under control and whose current EEGs are normal or near normal, may be tapered off therapy after being seizure-free for 2 years.

Children with the following characteristics may be tapered off of medications if they are seizure-free for 4 years:
• symptomatic partial seizures,
• persistently abnormal EEGs,
• moderate, generalized seizures,
• neurologic abnormalities on examination, or
• those who take a long time to get seizures under control.

What Are the Teratogenic Effects of These Drugs?

Pregnant women taking anti-seizure medications have a 2–3x greater risk of having an infant with abnormalities. The most common, major malformations are cleft lip/palate, neural tube defects (spina bifida), and cardiac anomalies. Valproate increases the risk of neural tube defect by 1.5% and carbamazepine by 0.5–1.0%. The neural tube defect risk can be decreased with folic acid intake before pregnancy. Generally, most recommend not using valproic acid or carbamazepine and limiting treatment to a single anticonvulsant if possible.

Minor anomalies include nail hypoplasia, hypertelorism, low-set ears, prominent lips, and nasal bridge abnormalities.

All this notwithstanding, a woman on seizure medications still has a 90–95% chance of having a healthy baby.

Also, almost all drugs cause or promote a hemorrhagic diathesis in newborns that may not be prevented by vitamin K at birth. Many recommend giving oral vitamin K phytonadione (20 mg/day) to pregnant women in the last month of pregnancy.

What about Breastfeeding?

Breastfeeding is not contraindicated and should not be discouraged. Most often, the only problems are with phenobarbital or primidone, which may cause poor sucking or excessive drowsiness.

NEONATAL SEIZURES

Neonatal seizures are different from those that occur in older children. The incidence is estimated to be 0.5–2/100 live births. In NICUs, the incidence is much higher, with nearly 10% having seizures.

Neonates can have seizures with or without EEG changes. Neonates also may have unusual movements or atypical features of seizures, such as jitteriness or tremor movements, which may be misidentified as seizures.

Seizures in neonates may have varied etiologies: *SEPSIS!*
• Perinatal complications: Particularly neonatal asphyxia in full-term infants and intraventricular hemorrhage in premature infants. Hypoxic-ischemic encephalopathy is the most common cause of seizures in the newborn.
• Intraventricular hemorrhage (IVH): This mainly affects premature infants, and they usually have focal or multi-focal clonic seizures.
• Hypoglycemia: In the term newborn, significant hypoglycemia is defined as having a glucose level < 30 mg/dL in the first 72 hours of life, 40 mg/dL thereafter. In preterms, < 20 mg/dL is the cutoff. The absolute effect of hypoglycemia is confounded by other factors, but most also treat all seizing infants with glucose.
• Hypocalcemia: In the newborn, this is defined as having a calcium level < 7.0 mg/dL in association with normal or high phosphorus. Most occur in the prenatal period in premature infants or those with perinatal disorders. Seizures usually are due to underlying brain damage, but hypocalcemia can exacerbate a coexisting seizure disorder.
• Infections: Infections of the CNS make up ~ 10% of etiologies for neonatal seizures. Every infant who has a seizure needs a lumbar puncture (LP) to rule out meningitis. Most infections are bacterial, with 1/3 viral in origin, including CMV, HSV, enterovirus, and rubella. Toxoplasmosis is a parasite that can cause seizures. Chorioretinitis suggests CMV or toxoplasmosis. EEG findings in herpes can be characteristic with PLEDS (periodic lateralizing epileptiform discharges) in older children but are not typically seen in infants. Of note, an HSV-PCR is the diagnostic study of choice for herpes encephalitis, although there is a significant false-negative rate. Intracranial calcifications may be seen in CMV or toxoplasmosis, but not until later in life.

notes

- Congenital malformations of the brain: Obviously, if the brain is not formed correctly—for example, in holoprosencephaly or anencephaly—then seizures are likely.
- Benign neonatal sleep myoclonus (non-epileptic): This is synchronous bilateral clonic activity during the early stages of sleep. The myoclonus is often confused with neonatal seizures. The episodes only occur during sleep and stop when the baby is awakened. No anticonvulsant therapy is indicated.
- Familial neonatal seizures: Benign, neonatal seizures have been described in some families. The condition appears to be autosomal dominant (AD), with the defect on the long arm of chromosome 20. The seizures are clonic and begin within the 1st week of life. EEGs taken at the time of the seizures show focal and generalized patterns; interictal EEGs are usually normal. No other findings occur. Usually the seizures eventually stop; however, 15% will develop epilepsy.

Before treatment for neonatal seizures, first identify a potential electrolyte abnormality and treat that quickly. The next step is to be sure that the infant is really having true seizures and not some other neurologic activity or event.

Treat infrequent or transient seizures with diazepam 0.1–0.5 mg IV, and repeat as needed. If seizures occur more often, or are more severe, give phenobarbital at 20 mg/kg IV, with a repeat dose as needed. A typical maintenance dose of phenobarbital is 3–5 mg/kg/day. If phenobarbital is not effective, you may give fosphenytoin 20 mg/kg slowly over 20 minutes, with ECG monitoring.

When to stop therapy? Most neonatal seizures will resolve by 1 month of age. Most pediatricians stop anti-seizure medications 1 month after the last seizure if the neurologic examination is normal. Some will not continue anti-seizure medications past 3 months, unless the EEG is significantly disturbed in the face of an abnormal neurologic examination.

FEBRILE SEIZURES

Febrile seizures occur in children ages 6 months–5 years. To meet the definition, there must not be intracranial infection or inflammation, and the child must not have experienced a prior seizure in the absence of fever. The febrile seizure is considered "simple" if the seizure lasts < 15 minutes, is non-focal, and does not recur during the same febrile illness. 80% meet these criteria for "simple." A "complex" febrile seizure has focal findings, longer duration, or recurs within 24 hours.

How common are these? Very! In some series, ~ 5% of children will experience at least one febrile seizure before 5 years of age. 50% of these will occur before 18 months of age. Risk factors include family history, attendance at daycare, and winter season. The majority of children with febrile seizures are developmentally and neurologically normal.

According to some texts and specialists, the likelihood for a febrile seizure is most often related to how rapidly the temperature rises, rather than the actual elevation of the temperature; however, this is still controversial and some think it is the actual elevation. Certain common infections, particularly roseola (human herpesvirus 6) and *Shigella* infection, result in a higher incidence of febrile seizures.

Family history is very important. ~ 40% of those affected will have at least one 1st or 2nd degree relative with a febrile seizure. In some families, the predilection is so strong that an AD mode of inheritance has been noted.

History and physical examination are very important to identify the focus of the fever, if possible, and to rule out other potential etiologies for the seizure. In young children, this often requires a lumbar puncture.

New practice parameters were being developed in late 2009 and may change the workup of febrile seizure. Currently, most recommend LP for those < 12 months. Most would also recommend LP in these situations:
- In the presence of meningeal signs and symptoms.
- In children 6–12 months of age in whom immunization status is unknown or in those who are non- or incompletely immunized.
- LP likely should be done in those who received antibiotics prior to their seizure.

Some lab work may be required, including electrolytes and glucose—if vomiting and diarrhea are part of the underlying illness—to determine whether an electrolyte abnormality is the etiology of the seizure.

What about CT or MRI? Consider these if the child has a complex febrile seizure, or especially if the child takes a long time to recover, or if he/she has a preexisting, undiagnosed neurologic or developmental abnormality.

What about EEG? It's pretty much useless in the evaluation of simple febrile seizures.

Do simple febrile seizures damage the brain? No. Most of these resolve very quickly and do not require special intervention. Ensure a clear airway and give oxygen, if available. Intubation is not necessary. Febrile status epilepticus is a whole different entity. These children may have brain damage from an attack that lasts > 30 minutes. Treat these children as though they have status epilepticus.

What about prevention of future febrile seizures? Do not give anti-seizure medications to children with simple febrile seizures, even if they recur. Many recommend giving those with fever antipyretics and tepid baths, but it has not been shown that these approaches actually prevent febrile seizures. For children with one or more prolonged attacks, or if the recurrences are very frequent, some recommend phenobarbital. However, this must be given with the caveat that this agent has long-term behavioral side effects. Some recent data support the use of valproate, but note: Although studies have shown that valproic acid is at least as effective as phenobarbital and significantly more effective than placebo in preventing febrile seizure recurrence, it should not be used because of the risk of hepatotoxicity in this age group (6 months to 5 years). Carbamazepine and phenytoin do not prevent recurrent febrile seizures. Rectal diazepam has been

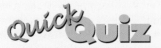

approved for use in children who have frequent febrile seizures and may be used by parents to abort attacks in those with recurrent prolonged attacks.

Who is at risk for recurrence?
Generally, children who have:
• their first seizure before age 18 months,
• a history of seizure with only a modest temperature elevation (< 40° C [104° F]), or
• suffered a seizure after having the fever for only a very short duration.
Note: Children whose first simple febrile seizure occurs when they are < 12–15 months have a 50% chance of recurrence.

About 65% of children with febrile seizures have only one episode. Of the 35% of children who experience a recurrence, 50% will have a second recurrence.

Approximately 2.5% of those children with simple febrile seizures will eventually develop epilepsy, but this is likely genetic in nature and not due to structural damage arising from the febrile seizures. Alternatively, as many as 50% of children who have had complex febrile seizures may develop temporal lobe epilepsy when they are older. It is not yet clear whether this is due to structural damage from the seizures or underlying mesial temporal sclerosis.

MIGRAINE HEADACHES

Migraine headaches are also discussed briefly in the Common Pediatric Disorders section.

Migraines were once thought to be due to vascular disturbances, but recent data suggest that they may actually be due to abnormalities with serotonin and other brain receptors. To meet the adult definition, migraines must occur at least 5 times and last 2–72 hours without an identifiable etiology. The patient must also report 2 of the following findings:
• Pain on one side
• Pulsating/throbbing character
• Moderate-to-severe intensity
• Increasing severity with activity

Additionally, the pain is usually associated with nausea, photophobia, and/or phonophobia. Often, younger children may not exhibit these characteristic features of adult migraines. Migraines can be spontaneous, induced by psychological stress, foods (chocolate [poor kids!], cheese, monosodium glutamate), or other factors. Auras are common in adults but relatively rare in children.

More unusual forms include:
• Hemiplegic migraine: The child has weakness on one side of the body with or without aphasia. This can last hours or even days! Some families have this with AD inheritance. This is different from alternating hemiplegia of childhood, which presents with paroxysmal, repeated episodes of hemiplegia lasting minutes to days, is associated with intellectual decline, and occurs in those < 18 months of age.
• Ophthalmoplegic migraine: An abnormality of eye movements. The 3rd cranial nerve is typically affected, and less commonly, the 4th or 6th cranial nerves may be involved.
• Basilar artery migraine: Occurs more commonly in adolescent girls and presents with vertigo, syncope, and dysarthria. Some also have visual alterations and loss of consciousness.
• Confusional migraine: Presents as a profoundly confused state that lasts for hours.

Treatment is two-pronged: Alleviate pain in acute attacks and prevent further attacks. Initially, treat individual attacks with acetaminophen or ibuprofen for acute pain. Nasal sumatriptan is now recommended for use in adolescents over age 18.

For chronic prevention, most data are anecdotal, but frequently used agents include cyproheptadine, valproate, topiramate, calcium-channel blockers, and amitriptyline. The Boards still may recommend the use of propranolol (1–2 mg/kg/day divided tid), but it is rarely used anymore.

Tension and other headaches are discussed under the "Common Pain Syndromes of Childhood" heading of the Common Pediatric Disorders section.

One question that comes up all the time on the Board exam is: When should you get a CT/MRI in a child with a headache? The answer:
• Recent school failure or behavioral change
• Abnormal neurologic signs
• Fall-off in growth
• Headache that awakens a child from sleep
• Early morning headache with increase in frequency and severity
• Headache with focal seizure
• Migraine headache, followed by a seizure

notes

- Headache associated with vomiting in the absence of a family history of migraine
- Cluster headaches in children
- Any child < 5 years with chief complaint of headache (controversial)
- Focal neurologic findings
- Brief coughing episode resulting in headache
- Increasing or "crescendo" headaches
- Persistent focal headaches
- Increase in head circumference
- Increase with Valsalva maneuvers

NEUROMUSCULAR DISEASES
SPINAL MUSCULAR ATROPHY

Spinal muscular atrophy (SMA) is the 2nd most common lethal autosomal recessive (AR) disorder! (Cystic fibrosis is #1.) The gene is located on chromosome 5q. Patients with spinal muscular atrophy present with hypotonia, weakness of the intracostal muscles, muscle atrophy, and fasciculations. The lesion responsible is degeneration of the anterior horn cell and, sometimes, also the bulbar nuclei. Muscle weakness is symmetric, with the proximal muscles affected to a greater degree. The legs are more affected than the arms. Because this affects only the motor anterior horn cell, no sensory or intellectual deficits are noted.

There are 3 types:
- Type I (Werdnig-Hoffman or severe infantile SMA): This is the most severe and presents at < 6 months of age with hypotonia and weakness, difficulty feeding, and tongue fasciculations. Most patients die by 2 years of age from respiratory failure.
- Type II (intermediate or chronic infantile SMA): Occurs in up to 1/15,000. Children appear healthy at birth and achieve initial normal milestones, but these are lost by 2 years of age. A majority die by age 12. Weakness can be static for long periods and then progresses with intercurrent illness.
- Type III (Kugelberg-Welder or mild SMA): This presents between ages 2 and 17 years, and the child becomes unable to walk or stand unaided. The degree of deficit correlates with the age of onset of symptoms.

Today, 95% can be diagnosed with gene mutation screening. CPK is normal. Management is aimed at aggressive respiratory, nutritional, and orthopedic interventions. Discuss with family the options of tracheostomy and lifelong mechanical ventilation before respiratory failure occurs.

DUCHENNE MUSCULAR DYSTROPHY

Duchenne muscular dystrophy is the most common form of muscular dystrophy. It occurs in ~ 1/3,000 male births and is an X-linked recessive disorder; thus the mother is a "carrier," but up to 30% of cases occur as spontaneous mutations. Duchenne's is caused by a mutation in the dystrophin gene and results in absent or deficient dystrophin protein.

Boys present between ages 2 and 6 years with frequent falling, a "waddling" gait, and toe walking. Classic things to look for on the Board exam: a child with calf muscle pseudohypertrophy and the Gowers sign—using arms to "climb up" the legs when rising from a seated position on the floor. CPK is elevated. Affected boys generally lose the ability to walk by 11 years of age. Respiratory muscle weakness corresponds to gross motor weakness. Eventually, he cannot handle respiratory secretions, and aspiration/infection commonly occurs. Cardiomyopathy is also a component of Duchenne's.

Diagnosis is made by either muscle biopsy, which will show missing or deficient dystrophin, or gene test.

Management is supportive. Scoliosis begins before loss of muscle function and progresses rapidly once the child is in a wheelchair. Long-term care is an issue, and respiratory failure is a common cause of death. There is evidence to support the use of prednisone to delay wheelchair use.

MYASTHENIA GRAVIS

Myasthenia gravis is rare in children but still is the most common primary disorder of neuromuscular transmission. With this disease, the postsynaptic receptors for acetylcholine are reduced in number, resulting in the postjunctional membrane being less sensitive to acetylcholine.

Neonatal myasthenia gravis occurs when the newborn is exposed to transplacental passage of maternal acetylcholine receptor antibodies. The neonate presents within 72 hours of birth with hypotonia, weak cry, difficulty feeding, facial weakness, and palpebral ptosis. Respiratory compromise occurs due to aspiration and progressive respiratory muscle weakness. Neonatal myasthenia resolves in 2–12 weeks after the antibodies clear.

Congenital myasthenia gravis is an AR disorder with variable age in onset. Those affected do not have circulating antibodies to the acetylcholine receptor.

Juvenile myasthenia gravis is an acquired autoimmune disorder and affects girls more than boys, usually after the age of 10 years. 80–90% of affected children have circulating autoantibodies to acetylcholine receptors. The disease progresses gradually, with worsening muscle weakness and respiratory compromise. Muscle weakness is exacerbated by repetitive muscle use. Ocular muscles are involved.

Diagnosis of myasthenia gravis is best achieved by the following maneuver: Give anticholinesterase medication, such as edrophonium (Tensilon® test) or neostigmine, and look for transient improvement. EMG, with repetitive-stimulation studies looking for electro-decrements, and/or serologic evaluation for the antibodies can also be helpful.

Treat with oral anticholinesterase medications; these can increase the concentration of acetylcholine at the receptor site. Immunosuppression can be beneficial as well. Thymectomy may induce remission in as many as 50–60%. Finally, plasmapheresis is beneficial for short-term amelioration of worsening symptoms.

notes

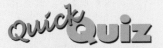

Quick Quiz

1) Describe Werdnig-Hoffman syndrome.
2) What is a common presentation for a boy with Duchenne muscular dystrophy?
3) How is Duchenne muscular dystrophy diagnosed?
4) How does juvenile myasthenia gravis present?
5) How is myasthenia gravis diagnosed?
6) How does Guillain-Barré syndrome classically present?
7) What is helpful about a lumbar puncture in Guillain-Barré syndrome?
8) How do infants with botulism present?
9) How do older children with botulism present? How are they treated?
10) What is acute cerebellar ataxia of childhood?
11) What is transverse myelitis?
12) How does multiple sclerosis present in childhood?

GUILLAIN-BARRÉ SYNDROME

Guillain-Barré syndrome (acute inflammatory demyelinating polyradiculoneuropathy) is a disorder that is traditionally presented on Board exams. Look for a child with acute paralysis, beginning with weakness of the legs, followed by increasing areas of paralysis moving upward toward the head. It can progress to involve the respiratory muscles and the cranial nerves. Sensory losses are rare and restricted to the vibratory and position sense. Tendon reflexes also are absent. The Babinski sign is not present. Less commonly, there can be autonomic instability, blood pressure problems (hypo- and hypertension), papilledema, and ataxia. Usually, bladder function is okay.

The etiology of Guillain-Barré is unknown, but it is classically associated with preceding infections in some instances, especially *Campylobacter* (up to 30% of cases), *Mycoplasma*, or EBV.

Lumbar puncture can be helpful and may show elevated protein levels as high as 100–150 mg/dL. Usually, the WBC in the spinal fluid is < 10 cells/µL. Nerve conduction studies show slowing and/or decreased amplitudes, depending on the subtype.

Differentials are tick paralysis, toxic neuropathies, porphyria, botulism, transverse myelitis, and poliomyelitis. Transverse myelitis can be distinguished from Guillain-Barré syndrome, even in the presence of spinal shock, because patients with Guillain-Barré will not have a sensory level.

Treatment is supportive since the condition resolves over time. Plasmapheresis and IVIG can improve recovery time. Steroids have not shown any benefit. Permanent sequelae can occur in ~ 15% of patients. Most recover within 3–4 weeks, and complete recovery is predicted by 6 months. Avoid anti-hypertensive medications due to the acute autonomic instability, which can induce severe hypotensive crisis.

BOTULISM

Botulism is due to the effects of *Clostridium botulinum* toxin. The toxin affects the presynaptic mechanisms that release acetylcholine in response to nerve stimulation; there is total paralysis of nicotinic and muscarinic cholinergic transmission. The toxin is produced by spores of the *Clostridium botulinum* and can contaminate soil-grown foods and fish. In the past, outbreaks occurred in infants given honey at very young ages. Recent outbreaks have occurred in commercial carrot juice and cheese sauce. The highest rates in the U.S. occur in Alaska and are due to ingestion of fermented fish.

Infants with botulism have constipation, generalized weakness, decreased ability to suck, poor gag reflexes, absence of deep tendon reflexes, facial diplegia, ptosis, and dry mouth. (See Figure 11-15—Note the complete lack of muscle tone and head control.) On the Board exam, look for a child with these findings and especially an infant with symmetrical findings, no drooling or secretions, dry mouth, and lack of pupillary response to light. Electrophysiologic testing will show an initial, very small, evoked-muscle action potential; but at high rates (20–50 Hz), the evoked response will be potentiated > 400%! For infants, look for the presence of *C. botulinum* in stool samples; the toxin can also be identified. Older children with food-borne botulism will likely have toxin identified in the blood as well.

Older children will have dryness and soreness of the mouth, blurry vision, double vision, nausea, and vomiting. They also will have a lack of sweating (anhidrosis), ophthalmoplegia, and symmetrical facial, bulbar, and limb abnormalities. The pupils are frequently paralyzed as well.

Admit all affected children to an ICU and carefully monitor for respiratory failure. Give antitoxin and guanidine, although guanidine is unproven in clinical trials. Infants are not routinely given these medications.

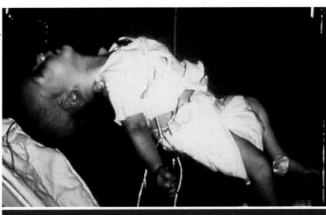

Figure 11-15: Child with Botulism Poisoning

notes

MISCELLANEOUS DISORDERS

NOTE

Note: All of the infectious diseases affecting the CNS (e.g., meningitis and encephalitis) are discussed in the Infectious Disease section. The neurometabolic and neurogenetic diseases are discussed in the Metabolic Disorders and Genetics sections, respectively.

ACUTE CEREBELLAR ATAXIA OF CHILDHOOD

Acute cerebellitis or acute cerebellar ataxia of childhood occurs most commonly in children ages 2–6 years. Its onset is abrupt, and about 50% of those affected have a history of prior URI or viral GI illness. These viruses can include varicella, rubeola, mumps, rubella, echoviruses, EBV, and influenza. Some bacterial infections, such as group A streptococcus and *Salmonella*, have also been implicated.

The ataxia can be mild or severe. Frequent findings include:
- Hypotonia
- Tremor
- Horizontal nystagmus
- Dysarthria

The child is irritable and has nausea/vomiting. The sensory exam is normal, as are the deep tendon reflexes. CSF is normal, except for an occasional increased WBC to 30 lymphocytes/μL. CT and MRI of the head are normal.

Around 90% recover without specific therapy in 6–8 weeks. Steroids are not indicated.

TRANSVERSE MYELITIS

Transverse myelitis refers to segmental spinal cord disease with both motor and sensory abnormalities at and below the level of the lesion. It also is associated with nonspecific viral infections. Most lesions occur at the thoracic cord level.

The illness begins with severe back pain that radiates around to the front. This is followed by rapidly progressive paraparesis, loss of sphincter tone, and loss of pain and temperature sensations below the level of the lesion. 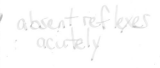 *absent reflexes acutely* MRI will frequently show an intramedullary signal change. CSF is generally normal or reveals mild pleocytosis and mild elevation in CSF protein—but evaluation should be done only after careful examination and consultation with a neurologist.

Prognosis is fairly good, with 60% having return of functional abilities and only 10–15% with permanent, severe damage. There is no specific therapy.

MULTIPLE SCLEROSIS

Multiple sclerosis (childhood demyelinating disease) is rare in childhood; only about 5% of patients with MS had their disease start < age 10 years. Most are affected in adolescence.

Symptoms mimic those in adults, with vision abnormalities, oculomotor disturbance, incoordination, and sensory deficits. On the Board exam, look for an adolescent with optic neuritis! All of the symptoms tend to remit and recur. CSF IgG or oligoclonal bands are increased in 75% of patients, but this finding is nonspecific. MRI is helpful in diagnosis and will show demyelination.

Treat acute exacerbations with short-term, high-dose, pulse IV steroids for 3–5 days. The disease course is extremely variable.